VISUAL DISPLAY TERMINALS
and
WORKERS' HEALTH

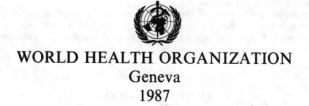

WORLD HEALTH ORGANIZATION
Geneva
1987

WHO Offset Publication No. 99

ISBN 92 4 170099 8

ISSN 0303-7878

PRINTED IN ENGLAND

87/7254-SB-7500

CONTENTS

Page

PREFACE   v

ACKNOWLEDGEMENTS   vi

1. EXECUTIVE SUMMARY   1

    1.1 Eye and visual problems   1
    1.2 Musculoskeletal disorders   1
    1.3 Stress related disorders   2
    1.4 Skin disorders   2
    1.5 Adverse reproductive outcomes   3

2. GENERAL INTRODUCTION   4

    2.1 Purpose and scope of this book   4
    2.2 Health issues in visual display terminal operations
         and the possible causal factors   5
    2.3 Research results and evaluation   6

3. GUIDELINES FOR WORK WITH VISUAL DISPLAY TERMINALS   10

    3.1 Introduction   10
    3.2 Intent and applicability of these recommendations   10
    3.3 Recommendations concerning the operator   11
    3.4 Recommendations concerning the visual display terminal .   12
    3.5 Recommendations concerning the workplace   12
    3.6 Recommendations concerning the work organization   13
    3.7 Recommendations concerning incidence of adverse health
         effects   14

4. ANSWERS TO SOME COMMON QUESTIONS ON HEALTH IMPLICATIONS
   OF WORK WITH VISUAL DISPLAY TERMINALS   15

5. BACKGROUND MATERIAL ON THE USE OF VISUAL DISPLAY TERMINALS . .   21

   5.1 Content   21
   5.2 Features of work on visual display terminals   22
        5.2.1 Description and classification of visual
               display terminals   22
        5.2.2 Electromagnetic radiation and fields from visual
               display terminals   27
               5.2.2.1 Potential electromagnetic radiations
                        and fields   31
               5.2.2.2 Ionizing radiation   32
               5.2.2.3 Optical radiation   34
               5.2.2.4 Hertzian radiation and fields   36
               5.2.2.5 Electrostatic fields   44
               5.2.2.6 Sound and noise from visual display
                        terminals   47
        5.2.3 Display characteristics and workroom lighting . .   48
               5.2.3.1 Time dependent variables of screen
                        luminants   48
               5.2.3.2 Structure of screen characters   54
               5.2.3.3 Luminance of screen information and
                        workroom lighting   55
        5.2.4 Work environment   62
               5.2.4.1 General physical characteristics . . .   63
               5.2.4.2 Physicochemical characteristics   64
               5.2.4.3 General factors for workstation design .   67
        5.2.5 Contextual factors   70
               5.2.5.1 Operator characteristics   72
               5.2.5.2 Job content   76
               5.2.5.3 Relationships between job content, work
                        environment and display utilization . . .   77
               5.2.5.4 Organizational conditions   80

5.3   Health considerations of work on visual display terminals   85

      5.3.1   Effects on the eyes and vision   85

              5.3.1.1   Asthenopia   86

              5.3.1.2   Correlations between eye discomfort and
                        other variables   88

              5.3.1.3   Studies on temporary changes in eye
                        functions   93

              5.3.1.4   Probable causes of discomfort among
                        VDT-operators   98

              5.3.1.5   Pathological changes in the eyes   103

      5.3.2   Musculoskeletal discomforts   108

              5.3.2.1   Occurrence of musculoskeletal symptoms .   109

              5.3.2.2   Correlations between musculoskeletal
                        symptoms and other variables   113

              5.3.2.3   Etiology of the observed musculoskeletal
                        complaints   116

              5.3.2.4   Repetitive motions and possible permanent
                        damage   118

      5.3.3   Headache   119

      5.3.4   Stress related disorders   122

              5.3.4.1   Psychological disturbances   123

              5.3.4.2   Behavioural consequences of work on
                        visual display terminals   124

              5.3.4.3   Physiological consequences of
                        psychosocial factors   125

              5.3.4.4   The possibility of persistent health
                        consequences   127

              5.3.4.5   Relations between stress disorders and
                        potential stress factors found during
                        work on visual display terminals   127

      5.3.5   Skin disorders   130

              5.3.5.1   Occurrence of skin disorders   131

              5.3.5.2   Possible causes of the skin disorders . .   133

      5.3.6   Photosensitive epilepsy   136

5.3.7   Adverse reproductive outcomes   137

       5.3.7.1   Reported clusters of spontaneous
abortions or congenital defects   138

       5.3.7.2   Statistical evaluation of reported
clusters   141

       5.3.7.3   VDT-related factors and adverse
reproductive outcomes   142

       5.3.7.4   The effects of extra-low-frequency
magnetic fields on chick embryogenesis .   143

       5.3.7.5   Research studies on pregnancy outcomes .   147

5.4   Recommendations for further research   158

   5.4.1   Concerning effects on the eyes and vision   158

   5.4.2   Concerning musculoskeletal disorders   159

   5.4.3   Concerning skin disorders   159

   5.4.4   Concerning stress factors and stress disorders . .   159

   5.4.5   Comments   160

REFERENCES   161

Annex 1.   List of participants in the WHO Working Group on
Occupational Health Aspects in the Use of Visual
Display Terminals.   192

Annex 2.   Visual Display Terminals of non-cathode
ray tube design.   194

Annex 3.   A model study on the occurrence of adverse
pregnancy outcomes in clusters of workers using
visual display terminals   201

PREFACE

Early awareness and rapid communication of findings pertaining to workers' health and safety problems are essential for the early detection and control of occupational hazards. The Workers Health Programme of the World Health Organization is making every effort to be responsive to this need.

Reports of potential health risks connected with the use of visual display terminals are of major concern to the millions of workers who use them as a part of their daily work activities. This technology is proliferating very rapidly, not only in industrialized countries, but in developing countries as well.

In the wake of this expanding use of visual display terminals and the expressed concern about adverse health effects among visual display terminal operators, the World Health Organization asked Dr Ulf OV. Bergqvist and Professor Bengt Knave, of the National Board of Occupational Health and Safety in Sweden, to prepare a review of information bearing on this problem and to evaluate it critically. This document was circulated to the WHO Collaborating Centres for Occupational Health for review and comment prior to a meeting of a Working Group on Occupational Health Aspects in the Use of Visual Display Terminals that was held in Geneva on 2-6 December 1985.[1] The manuscript was finalized after this meeting and is published in the hope that it will facilitate the transfer of technical information not otherwise readily available to those responsible for improving workers' health.

---

[1] The participants in this meeting are listed in Annex 1.

ACKNOWLEDGEMENTS

The World Health Organization is pleased to acknowledge the valuable comments on the background document that were provided by the WHO Collaborating Centres for Occupational Health; the Working Group found them most helpful in their discussions. The World Health Organization also gratefully acknowledges the permission granted by the Editor of the Scandinavian Journal of Work, Environment and Health to reproduce information from a paper by Ulf OV. Bergqvist on video display terminals and health and that was published in that journal. Financial support for the work of Dr. Bergqvist was provided to the National Board of Occupational Safety and Health in Sweden by the Nordic Council of Ministers.

Technical and financial support provided to the WHO Workers Health Programme, under a cooperative agreement with the National Institute for Occupational Safety and Health, United States of America, a WHO Collaborating Centre for Occupational Health, is also gratefully acknowledged.

The special comments of Dr P. J. Waight, Division of Environmental Health, WHO, in the field of radiation exposures are gratefully acknowledged.

1. EXECUTIVE SUMMARY

A World Health Organization Working Group on Aspects of Occupational Health in the Use of Visual Display Terminals (VDTs) studied in December 1985 the considerable literature available from research that is pertinent to the health implications of work on VDTs. On the basis of these considerations, the working group arrived at the conclusions that are set out below.

1.1 Eye and visual problems

Many reports have testified to the problems of eye discomfort of VDT-operators. Concern has also been voiced about the possibility that damage to the visual system may occur as a result of working with VDTs.

The working group concluded that visual system discomfort was a common problem when working with VDTs. The group concluded, however, that there was no evidence of damage or permanent impairment to the visual system of persons working with VDTs. Further research including longitudinal studies is underway. The working group wished to emphasize, however, that the visual discomfort occurring in those working with VDTs must be recognized as a health problem. It was the working group's conclusion that such discomfort is largely avoidable. The group emphasized that attention should be given to design of the equipment, the workplace, the work environment and to work practices to prevent eye discomfort. The group also felt that attending to the visual health needs of workers using VDTs is essential to an effective preventive approach.

1.2 Musculoskeletal disorders

Reports of occurrences of musculoskeletal discomfort are frequent among users of VDTs. The possibility of long-term effects resulting from such discomfort has also been discussed.

The working group recognized that musculoskeletal discomfort was commonplace during work with VDTs. Injury from repeated stress to the musculoskeletal system is possible; such effects have been observed in other jobs. Further research on the potential for injury is warranted. However, the group emphasized that these conclusions should not be interpreted to mean that musculoskeletal discomfort inevitably leads to injury or is necessarily a sign of injury. It was the view of the working group that musculoskeletal problems in work associated with VDTs are largely preventable and that appropriate control measures should be introduced. These include the application of ergonomic principles to the design of the workplace equipment, to the environment and to work organization. Occupational health services play a key role in the early recognition and prevention of musculoskeletal problems in persons using VDTs.

1.3 Stress related disorders

Stress factors and stress-related disorders have been repeatedly discussed in relation to work with VDTs. Arguments as to the role of the VDT system itself, as compared with the role of other factors such as job design and organization have been put forward.

Many aspects of working conditions can lead to stress-related disorders; these are referred to as stress factors. The working group found little consistent evidence of abnormal levels of stress-related disorders (either physical, psychological, or behavioural) among workers using VDTs. However, the group noted considerable evidence that stress factors associated with that work may create health problems. The working group concluded that additional research is warranted to investigate stress disorders among such workers. The group recognized that certain intervention and control strategies could improve working conditions with respect to stress factors and urged their implementation.

1.4 Skin disorders

Indications of certain skin disorders among operators of VDTs have occurred in some countries. The amount of scientific data on this point is still rather limited.

The working group considered reports of skin disorders in a number of VDT operators. The most frequently reported are non-specific facial skin rashes and aggravation of rosacea (a facial condition marked by flushing, red coloration and acne-like appearance of the skin). The working group was also aware of the case of a Swedish VDT operator with a skin disorder, diagnosed as elastosis solaris (premature aging of the skin), which had been recognized by a worker's compensation board in Sweden as a work-related disease. The cause of these skin disorders is not clear. Further research is essential on the issue of skin disorders and working on VDTs.

1.5 Adverse reproductive outcomes

The appearance of clusters of spontaneous abortions among VDT operators, or of congenital defects in their children, has led to widespread concern about the possibility of a relationship between work with VDTs and adverse effects on pregnancy.

The working group considered the issue of potential adverse pregnancy outcomes associated with the use of VDTs. The working group was aware of a number of studies in progress, the results of which will be evaluated when they become available. Recent studies were examined and the group concluded that those studies provide no evidence of a link between adverse effects on pregnancy and the use of VDTs. This should not be interpreted, however, to mean that working on VDTs is absolutely safe. Measures are advisable, however, to avoid excessive discomfort and fatigue for a pregnant woman who is using the VDT.

2. GENERAL INTRODUCTION

2.1 Purpose and scope of this book

Visual display terminals (VDTs) are used by millions of workers throughout the world, as a part of their daily activities. This technology is proliferating very rapidly, not only in industrialized countries, but in developing countries as well.

In the wake of this expanding use of VDTs, concern has been expressed and reports have appeared about adverse health effects among VDT operators. Earlier, this concern was largely directed towards ergonomic aspects – primarily of vision – in Europe, and the possibility of radiation hazards in North America. Health effects that have been considered include eye problems (both discomfort and damage), musculoskeletal pain, headache, stress disorders, skin disorders, and miscarriages or birth defects. In recent years, our knowledge on these possible effects has expanded and in part has been consolidated, making conclusions possible on many of the issues.

Organization of the publication

The working group realized that the conclusions they arrived at should be made available to a wide variety of readers – workers using VDTs, employers, trade union representatives, and occupational health workers as well as research workers in that field.

The need to present the rather voluminous data that exist, has resulted in a rather long book. In order to make it easier for readers to find the information they require, condensed conclusions and evaluations are provided in the following sections:

- The executive summary (pp. 1 – 3) provides precise and condensed statements from the working group – summarizing their evaluation of the data on the major possible health implications of the use of VDTs. Readers who wish to study the data on which these evaluations are made are referred to the appropriate parts of Section 5.3.

- Readers requiring some guidelines on VDT workstations and VDT work arrangements, will find these on pages 10 - 14. Those guidelines are intended to prevent known, or clearly indicated, adverse effects which are related to the use of VDTs.

- A number of questions are often raised concerning possible health risks associated with the use of VDTs. On pages 15 - 20, the working group has attempted to phrase and answer those questions that are met most frequently. After each question, the reader is given references to appropriate parts of Section 5 - the background material.

The remainder of the book consists of background material, where the detailed data used by the working group is described. The background material also contains some recommendations for further research, on areas where the group recognized insufficiencies in knowledge on the health implications of work with VDTs.

2.2 Health issues in visual display terminal operations and the possible causal factors

Health is defined in the Constitution of the World Health Organization not only as an absence of disease or infirmity, but also as a state of complete physical and mental and social well-being. This definition of health forms the basis for the evaluations made by the working group. Specifically, the group emphasizes that various types of discomfort must be considered as health problems. The focus of this report, as well as a major part of the background data, is related to the use of VDTs in office work, but many parts of the report are also applicable to the use of VDTs in other contexts.

It should also be emphasized that all adverse health effects occurring in VDT workers, as in other workers, should be taken seriously, regardless of the cause. In this publication, however, the working group was concerned with whether the appearance or aggravation of health problems was directly related to the use of visual display terminals, since any indication or confirmation of such a relationship would provide the basis for measures to prevent the adverse effects.

In view of the ongoing concern in Europe on the health aspects of visual display terminals, the WHO Regional Office for Europe has organized a scientific review of the subject[1].

Different work factors in relation to visual display terminals

While there is, by and large, a fairly good understanding of the different health problems associated with the use of VDTs, knowledge of the specific causal factors that may be involved is more limited. It is the working group's understanding that health effects of work with VDTs are caused by a number of interrelated factors.

Various proposals have been made for a single factor that would explain all the reported (or suggested) health effects of working with VDTs. The two extremes of these proposals are as follows: in one, a specific radiation factor is held to be the cause, while in the other, all the adverse health effects are considered to be due to the negative attitude of VDT operators towards their work. Research data do not give credibility to either of these suggestions. The working group again wished to emphasize that health effects of work with VDTs result from many causes.

The group considered two different types of possible factors. One type is concerned with the physical aspects of the VDT and the working environment, while the other includes the job content, and the organization of work, as well as other psychosocial factors. For many effects, e.g., eye discomfort, a full understanding of causes can only be arrived at by combining various factors of the two types.

In addition, individual factors such as age, existing disorders, or individual sensitivity may influence the appearance or manifestation of different adverse health effects.

2.3 Research results and evaluation

The presented evaluation of possible health effects of working with VDTs is based on existing and available knowledge. Future research results may, of course, result in the modification or confirmation of conclusions made here, or may clarify areas for which no conclusions can at present be made.

---

[1] Marriott, I.A. & Studily, M.A. (In preparation).

The working group, when discussing a specific issue, had to consider first whether there were sufficient data on which to base any conclusion; if so, then they deliberated on what conclusion could be made. In this context, the working group wishes to emphasize, that a recommendation for further research studies on an issue should not be taken to imply that at present it is impossible to reach a conclusion on that issue.

Types of research investigations

Awareness of the possibility of a problem has primarily come from reports on cases of occurrences of adverse health effects among VDT-operators. A special form of this is the appearance of "clusters" of cases, these having been observed primarily in relation to adverse reproductive effects. Reports on cases and clusters are invaluable for initiating research. Investigations of cases or clusters may also provide valuable suggestions regarding the factors to be investigated. The working group wishes to emphasize, however, that conclusions valid for other groups cannot be made only on the basis of cases or cluster appearances.

Results from experimental research are valuable in considering which factors may be involved. In general, there is a fruitful interaction between experimental research and epidemiological studies in this respect.

Epidemiological studies are a particularly important aspect of research in this field. In this respect, however, the nature of VDT work does pose difficulties - since a number of contributing and conflicting factors must be considered. Some of these problems will be discussed below.

The working group's evaluation of the health risks associated with the use of VDTs was, whenever possible, made on the combined evidence from experimental research evaluation and from the results of epidemiological studies. When a number of reliable epidemiological studies were available, the evaluation was based mainly on these; this was the case as regards the issues of eye discomfort, musculoskeletal discomfort, and adverse reproductive outcomes.

For some other issues, e.g., cataract formation and stress disorders, the evaluations relied to a larger degree on a knowledge of whether VDT work involved any known risk factors for these problems.

Some comments on epidemiological studies

It is evident that the quality of the reports on epidemiological studies is very varied. When evaluating these studies, a number of problems were considered by the working group, e.g., the size and the statistical power of the study, administrative aspects of questionnaire responses, the response rate, the methods and results of statistical analysis - including analyses to evaluate the influence of confounding or contributing factors, possibility of bias, etc.

The working group has explicitly reported details on this in three areas where it was considered essential to the reliability of the evaluation, namely, on eye damage, skin disorders, and adverse reproductive outcome.

Some comments on terminology

In many reports or discussions, ambiguous terms are used that may lead to problems of interpretation. Some examples are mentioned here; however, the reader is referred to Section 5 for further discussion of these matters:

-   Eye discomfort: the term asthenopia has also been used, as defined on page 85. Other uses of this term occur, however. The term eye strain is also used in many reports.

-   Repetitive strain injury: this term has been used in some reports to imply organic damage. However, the term is utilized in other reports reviewed and refers only to muscle discomfort and pain (see p. 118). A precise definition is recommended in this report.

-   Stress: the terms stress factors and stress-related disorders are used as described on pages 122 and 123.

-   Congenital malformation: this term is sometimes used to imply any malformation and sometimes to mean significant malformation (see p. 138).

-   Polarity: in the present context, a positive polarity screen means dark characters on bright background, with negative polarity meaning the opposite.

Other ambiguities are discussed in the text where appropriate. The
working group also wishes to emphasize the need for specific and clearly
defined diagnoses in further studies. In addition, the group feels that the
term "VDT-exposed" is somewhat misleading, since it gives the impression that,
as regards health effects, the VDT should be regarded as a single factor. The
dichotomy of "VDT-exposed" versus "non-VDT" may be inappropriate in many
respects, especially concerning stress-related disorders.

3. GUIDELINES FOR WORK WITH VISUAL DISPLAY TERMINALS

3.1 Introduction

The increased use of visual display terminals in many types of workplace
has drawn attention to a number of adverse health effects which are, or are
alleged to be, caused by working with VDTs. Research has confirmed that the
increased occurrence of certain kinds of discomfort is related to the use of
VDTs, while other alleged health effects do not appear to be related to VDT
use.

These guidelines are intended to provide advice for the prevention of
those adverse effects that have been shown to be, or do appear to be, related
to the use of VDTs. It should be recognized, that the scientific basis for
these recommendations is restricted to currently known data. Modifications of
statements made here may thus become necessary, if new data appear.
Nevertheless, statements made in these recommendations are based on fairly
extensive evidence.

The recommendations are structured according to (a) the type of factor
involved, and (b) the aspect of the work or the equipment that might be
modified in order to decrease the occurrence of the adverse effects. The
different sections thus concern the operator, the VDT unit, the workplace, and
the organization of work, respectively.

3.2 Intent and applicability of these recommendations

Intent of these recommendations

These recommendations are intended to ensure (as far as possible) that
visual display terminals, and work performed with these terminals, should be
so designed that no individual should develop adverse health effects as a
result of VDT work.

Applicability of these recommendations - the visual display terminal

These recommendations concern work being performed using a visual display
terminal - a device for the visual presentation of electronically stored
information. They do not concern work with oscilloscopes, radar or with

displays of measuring instruments, etc., although certain sections may also serve as a guide for work with these devices.

Most of the knowledge upon which these recommendations are based, is derived from situations where VDTs based on a cathode ray tube were used. Nevertheless, these recommendations should, for the present, also be considered applicable to the use of VDTs based on other techniques such as plasma, electroluminescent or liquid crystal displays.

Applicability of these recommendations - the work performed

The recommendations are applicable to work situations where the use of visual display terminals forms a significant part of the work.

Applicability of these recommendations - the effects

The recommendations are intended as protection against those adverse health effects that may be associated with the use of VDTs.

3.3 Recommendations concerning the operator

General recommendations

It is intended that no invidual should be excluded from working on VDTs, except on the basis of insurmountable disabilities.

There are at present no indications that work with VDTs causes photosensitive epileptic seizures. Nevertheless, persons known to be susceptible to photosensitive epileptic seizures should consult a physician before commencing VDT work.

Should a pregnant woman show great concern and worry about working with a VDT, this worry must be taken seriously, although it may be explicitly stated that the worry is not justified on the basis of scientific evidence. Decisions - on an individual basis - for alternative work because of this worry may, however, be advisable.

Eye examination

Certain eye conditions such as presbyopia may contribute to the development of eye and musculoskeletal discomfort during VDT work. Therefore, operators should undergo an eye examination before starting to work with a VDT, and also at least every fifth year after the age of 40 years. These examinations should be performed by qualified personnel and should include refraction, visual acuity and when necessary prescriptions for new glasses required for near work (near additions). The examinations should be related to the operator's specific working conditions. VDT workers should be made aware of the fact that these examinations are not a substitute for complete visual health care.

3.4 Recommendations concerning the visual display terminal

Visual ergonomics

Low display quality and readability appear to be important factors for visual discomfort, and probably also for muscle discomfort. The characteristics of the display are affected by a number of specifications, concerning the structure, the luminance and the time appearance of the picture elements (dots/strokes) and the formed characters. National and international organizations have issued recommendations on these points. The International Organization for Standardization is currently developing standards for visual ergonomic characteristics of VDTs.

System design

Particular attention must be given to the operational aspects of the VDT system, including software, as these can play a role as stress factors.

3.5 Recommendations concerning the workplace

Lighting affects visual ergonomics. The introduction of a VDT into a workplace may necessitate several lighting adjustments. The workplace should be arranged in such a way that glare and reflections do not occur, particularly on the work surfaces, including the keyboard and the keys.

However, the use of antireflection devices should not interfere with the
display image quality. Thus, the use of additional filters may not be
advisable - unless reflections cannot be prevented or eliminated in any other
way.

The ambient lighting level must be appropriate to the task, to the
readability of both the VDT display and the manuscript, as well as to the
individual's sensitivity. Screens with dark characters on a light background
may require less modification of the workplace lighting than screens with
light characters on a dark background. To read manuscripts, some people may
require a separate adjustable task light. Large differences in luminance in
the field of vision, and between different areas of visual work, should be
avoided.

Design of the work station

The design of the work station is important in order to avoid muscle
discomfort. The primary objectives are to ensure that the positions of
keyboard, screen, manuscript holder, etc., are fully adjustable to the
preferences of the individual operator. Keyboards should be thin and
detachable.

Work environment

Excessive heat in VDT workplaces may cause discomfort problems and should
be eliminated. In addition, noise output from VDTs should be minimized and
excessive electrostatic charges should be eliminated.

3.6 Recommendations concerning the organization of work

Time restrictions for work with visual display terminals

The types of work performed at VDTs differ in many important respects,
among them the length of time spent actually looking at the screen; this
clearly affects the importance of the quality of the display in relation to
the working conditions. In consequence, it does not appear feasible to assign
general rules as to the length of time spent working with a VDT. It should,
however, be emphasized that it may be possible to establish time limits for
VDT work in particular situations.

Work breaks are important in order to avoid discomfort. The types of breaks can be varied, however, both longer breaks and short pauses being important. The frequency of breaks should be adjusted to the type and intensity of the work performed.

Intensive use of visual display units

Adverse effects are most commonly associated with strictly regimented, constrained, and monotonous routine work. Measures should be taken to improve such jobs.

Introduction of visual display terminals

The reaction of the staff to the introduction of VDTs is partly dependent on the provision of information and the participation of the staff in the planning, design, and implementation stages. Adequate training is also essential.

3.7 Recommendations concerning the incidence of adverse health effects

The first step should be to examine whether the VDT, the workplace, and the work organization are in accordance with the recommendations given and to ensure that appropriate adjustments are carried out. Should problems persist, the individual should be referred for an appropriate medical consultation.

4. ANSWERS TO SOME COMMON QUESTIONS ON THE HEALTH IMPLICATIONS
    OF WORK WITH VISUAL DISPLAY TERMINALS

a) Are there health risks associated with VDT work?

Adverse health effects include discomfort, and, in this sense, there are
certainly health risks associated with working with VDTs. In general,
most health problems appear to be similar to those encountered in more
traditional office work, although VDT work aggravates some of these. This
does not imply that concern over such problems should be ignored;
discomfort can be intense and a large number of individuals are affected.
Furthermore, many of these discomfort problems can be prevented,
eliminated or diminished by known control measures.

(See pp. 85-92; 108-116; 119-130).

b) What are the discomfort problems?

Discomfort generally occurs in the visual system (tired or irritated eyes,
etc.) or in the musculoskeletal system (particularly in the shoulder,
neck, and upper back region). VDT users as a whole do not appear to
suffer unusual levels of psychosocial stress or emotional problems,
although research points to instances of very demanding, stressful work on
VDTs, where such problems may be of concern.

(See pp. 85-92; 108-116; 119-130)

c) Are there particular problems for pregnant women?

There is no evidence that working with VDTs results in any adverse effects
on the outcome of pregnancy; worries about radiation are not based on
currently known facts. Nevertheless, measures are advisable to avoid
excessive discomfort and fatigue for a pregnant woman who is using the
VDT, by ensuring that she can sit comfortably, has good working
conditions, and is able to take regular breaks.

(See pp. 137-158)

d)   **Can work with VDTs affect the eyes/vision?**

There are no indications that work with VDTs will cause disease or damage
to the eyes. However, symptoms of discomfort are common when working with
a VDT, and can be disabling. Existing visual disorders or vision status
may influence any discomfort noticed during work on VDTs. These symptoms,
although, they appear to be transitory, should not be ignored. Control
measures include attention to lens prescriptions, to lighting and interior
design, and optimal design of the display (VDT and paper).

(See pp. 85-108)

e)   **Can work with VDTs cause musculoskeletal disorders?**

VDT work may cause musculoskeletal discomfort due to static efforts,
awkward posture, or highly repetitive tasks. Long-term damage appears
much less likely, although stereotyped motions during VDT work (as in
other desk work) may lead to chronic problems. Control measures include
attention to the design of tables and chairs, the display, keyboard and
document holders, as well as to the organization of work and the
diversification of tasks.

(See pp. 108-119)

f)   **Can working with a VDT cause skin or dermatological disorders?**

Some people seem to have had existing disorders aggravated or have
experienced skin rashes as a result of working with a VDT. Whether this
was due to the VDT itself or to other factors is not known. There is some
evidence that a combination of dry air, the electrostatic charge of the
operator, and individual susceptibility may be important factors - for at
least some of the reported cases - since increasing the humidity and
eliminating the static charge of the operator seem to help.

(See pp. 130-136)

- 17 -

g) <u>Is work with VDTs stressful?</u>

This kind of work is stressful in several respects - but many other types
of work can be equally stressful. One important point is that while the
concern is often centred on the VDT, the increased pace of work may be a
more important factor in many organizations. Some VDT workers may
experience less stress because the VDT gives them access to information
which they previously had to guess, while others may experience increased
stress because of the reliance on a system that may not function well, or
because of monitoring possibilities.

(See pp. 122-130)

h) <u>Are the health effects that have been noted temporary or permanent?</u>

Basically, they are temporary, and should recede after a short rest.
Discomfort persisting for several days after VDT work may signal a more
serious problem and is cause for a medical follow-up. Short-term
discomfort that occurs persistently during VDT work is a signal for
reconsidering the VDT-work situations (display, work environment, work
organization) and for a vision check.

(See pp. 86-88; 92-93; 96-97; 103-108; 108-111; 114-115; 118-119; 123-127;
131-133; 137-147)

i) <u>Can older workers use VDTs?</u>

Yes, but some extra precautions are called for - because of changes that
occur in the visual and musculoskeletal systems with aging. For example,
better working conditions are needed because of increased susceptibility
to some adverse visual conditions (glare, low contrast). The decrease in
accommodation capacity, which is normally compensated for by the use of
reading glasses, must be met by special glasses adjusted to the actual
reading distance. Workstation design and configuration as well as the
organiation of work may also have to be adjusted. Older people may also
need longer to get adjusted to work with VDTs.

(See pp. 73-74)

j)   How long can I work with VDTs (without problems)?

The maximum length of time an individual should work at a VDT is
variable. It depends on the operator, the task, how well the equipment
and environment are designed, and the mix of activities in the job. The
most effective mix is when people can choose to organize the work and take
small informal breaks rather than a rigid pattern of breaks. Such
minibreaks (of a few seconds duration) should probably be very frequent,
while longer breaks are often advisable after one or two hours - depending
on the job. The development of discomfort is a sign that counter measures
are needed - such measures may include changing the pattern of work.

(See pp. 80-81)

k)   Why do so many people complain about VDT work?

For a variety of reasons, such as: i) a growing awareness of the
importance of public health; ii) the fact that although the discomfort
may be minor compared to other health effects, it is nevertheless a
reality for a large proportion of those using VDTs; iii) an explosive
increase in VDT use throughout the world; iv) intense attention to this
problem by the media, and v) because VDTs are often the only visible part
of major changes occurring in work practices, and their use is often
accompanied by a "loss of control".

l)   Do VDTs emit hazardous levels of radiation?

No; in general the levels of electromagnetic radiation and the fields
found around VDTs are either nondetectable or insignificant compared with
the recognized hazard threshold. A detailed investigation has been
necessary for two field types; low-frequency pulsed magnetic fields and
electrostatic fields, which have been discussed in connection with adverse
effects on pregnancy and skin disorders, respectively. Studies to date
have, however, failed to show any relevant effects of the fields found
around VDTs.

(See pp. 27-48)

m) How important is maintenance?

Maintenance is very important, and includes considerations such as display legibility - which requires a clear and clean screen surface. The phosphor coating on the screen will deteriorate eventually, and this will be manifested as a decreased display quality. System malfunctions should be prevented, since unreliability in this respect is a known stress factor in many job situations. There are, however, no data to support the suggestions made that any malfunction could cause the emission of dangerous levels of ionizing radiation.

n) Are there product alternatives and how do we choose?

There are many ergonomically high quality products on the market - just as there are those of lower qualities. The exact product to choose depends on the work to be performed; alternative products (VDTs, etc.) should be tested in the actual work setting. Most VDTs are based on cathode ray tubes, although VDTs based on other techniques are available on the market. In general and for the present, the best choice for prolonged work is a high quality VDT based on a cathode ray tube.

(See Annex 2)

o) How important are these health concerns compared with those of other kinds of work, e.g., in industry or traditional office work?

Most of the problems seen in connection with VDT work will also be found in much traditional office work, although the introduction of the VDT may have aggravated some of them (e.g., eye discomfort). Control principles should also be somewhat similar. Compared with many industrial work situations, the health consequences discussed here are minor, but since they concern a very large number of people, often occur with a relatively high frequency (high risk) and are by and large avoidable, they cannot be considered unimportant.

p) <u>Is training needed, and where can I obtain more information?</u>

Training is definitely needed on all aspects of office work when
introducing and using VDTs. A major part of this training is relevant at
the time of introduction of VDTs (with follow-up training some time
later). Information materials include this publication, the International
Trade Union Guidelines, Conditions of Work Digest on VDTs (ILO), the
European Computer Manufacturers Association Technical Report, many
national documents, books and reports.

5. BACKGROUND INFORMATION ON THE USE OF VISUAL DISPLAY TERMINALS

5.1. Content

This review of background information commences with a brief discussion of
VDT technology, with the emphasis on cathode ray tube-based VDTs. Following
this, the different features of VDT work are discussed, which are of
importance when evaluating the possibility of health implications. These
features include electromagnetic radiation and fields, noise, display
characteristics, workroom lighting, the workstation and work environment as
well as the context of the use of VDTs. The latter includes operator
characteristics and job descriptions as well as psychosocial factors. A
review of the discussed implications of working on VDTs is then given; eye
problems, musculoskeletal discomforts, headache, stress disorders, skin
disorders, photosensitive epilepsy and adverse effects on reproduction.
Recommendations for further research are also presented. A brief description
and a discussion on other VDT techniques (e.g. plasma or liquid crystal) are
given in Annex 2, while some details of the evaluation of clusters of adverse
effects on pregnancies are to be found in Annex 3.

Data used for this report

The sources for data have been found by several methods. A number of data
based literature searches were made (in Medlars, Excerpta Medica, Pascal,
Health & Safety, Golem, Inspec, National Technical Information Service, Alcdok
and Serix). Further sources were International Labour Office bibliographies,
VDT News, Microwaves News etc. In addition, data were found by back
references in various reports, in conference proceedings and by personal
contacts. A further recent source of information concerning VDTs and health
has been furnished by the international scientific conference on work with
display units which was held in Stockholm, 12-15 May 1986. A number of the
findings presented at that conference were reviewed by the WHO working group
and have been included in the present publication.

The literature base is not restricted to published articles in scientific
journals. It also includes some unpublished or unreviewed reports in an effort
to give a comprehensive coverage of the subject.

5.2 Features of work on visual display terminals

5.2.1 Description and classification of visual display terminals

Description. A visual display terminal (VDT, sometimes called a visual
display unit, or video display unit, VDU), is a device for the visual
presentation of electronically stored information. It comprises a display
screen with a processing unit for information presentation and a keyboard for
control functions and data input. The unit may be separate, or connected to
other devices (e.g. computers). By definition, the "VDT concept" does not
include television sets, oscilloscopes, etc.

Classifications. Classification of VDTs pertinent to the discussion of
health effects is preferably based on construction principles and on certain
display parameters (e.g. multicolour capability, positive or negative
polarity, size etc.). Terms such as 'data input', 'interactive' etc. are
better applied to jobs performed at VDTs - a specific VDT design may be used
for a variety of purposes.

VDTs are normally based on cathode ray tubes (CRTs), and the screens are
then basically similar to television screens (see further below). VDTs based
on other techniques such as plasma or liquid crystal displays do exist, but
are as yet infrequent compared to CRT-based VDTs. (These are discussed in
Annex 2.)

Cathode ray tube-based visual display terminals. A cathode ray tube is
constructed according to the same general principles regardless of its
application; a television set or a VDT, etc. The major components are (see
Fig. 1):

A cathode serving as the electron source.

A grid, used to modulate the intensity of the electron beam. The electron
beam can be cut off by a sufficient increase in the potential difference
between the grid and the cathode (the grid being negative to the cathode).
Grid potentials are typically - 10 to - 100 volts.

A series of two to three <u>anodes</u> which accelerate and focus the electron beam. Focusing (and also some modulation) of the beam is achieved by varying the individual anode potentials (typically at a few hundred to a few thousand volts positive compared to the grid).

<u>Deflecting devices</u>, regulating the impact area on the screen. This is normally accomplished by an arrangement of magnetic coils outside of the tube. The trajectory of the beam depends on the magnetic fields induced by the coils; malfunctioning may result in aberrations or distortions of the beam shape etc. Electric deflection devices occur in other CRT applications (e.g. oscilloscopes), but rarely in VDT applications.

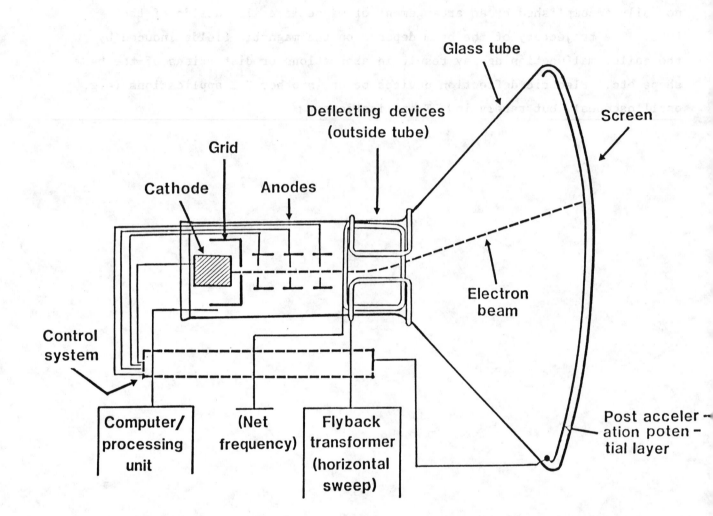

Fig. 1. The principle of CRT/VDT design

A CRT <u>screen</u>, consisting of two layers; first a metal layer given a high potential (post-acceleration potential) of up to approximately + 25 kV. Screens for colour applications, VDTs or television sets, have a higher voltage than monochromatic screens. This potential accelerates the electrons in the latter part of the trajectory. The layer also reflects light from the phosphor towards the observer, thus increasing the brightness of the screen image. Outside this metal layer is a fluorescent screen material, 'phosphor', where the electron energy is converted to light. This phosphor is in principle composed of a mineral (base) with a small amount of an activating (metal) material.

A <u>glass envelope</u> made conductive and with a permalloy layer, to shield the tube from electrostatic and magnetic fields.

The tube is sealed off to maintain a <u>vacuum</u> of some 10^{-4} Pa. Precautions are also taken against residual gas and ions produced within the tube.

<u>Application of the cathode ray tube to visual display terminal-operation</u>. The generation of text or a picture on the screen is dependent on some cyclic electromagnetic processes.

1. A saw-tooth magnetic field with a periodicity (refresh rate) of between about 50 and 100 Hz is applied to the vertical deflector system. This field gradually lowers the electron beam 'down' the screen, and then quickly returns the beam to the upper limit of the screen. This frequency normally corresponds to the refresh rate of the screen information. For a comment on interlace, see process 4 below.

2. A second saw-tooth magnetic field ('fly-back') gradually moves the beam towards the right of the screen, and then quickly returns the beam to the far left. This field, with a normal frequency of between 15 and 25 kHz is generated by the current from the fly-back transformer, and is applied to the horizontal deflecting system.

3. Modulation of the electron beam intensity in order to produce light or dark spots along the horizontal sweep. The maximum rate of on/off signals corresponds to the frequency of 'pixel' (picture element) generation, and is

usually performed with a digital clock frequency of the order of 5-10 MHz. The external signal from the computer or the processing unit (keyboard etc.) is applied to the gate, and the resultant grid potential can then cut off the electron beam, producing a dark spot.

4. Interlace implies that each line is refreshed only every second cycle. Thus, the refresh rate of each picture element is only 25 Hz for a 50 Hz refresh rate. The interlace technique is used in television sets, while its use in VDTs is less common (IBM, 1984).

The two 'fixed' (1 and 2) and one 'varied' signal (3) must be correlated in order to avoid distortions and unwanted lines when returning the beam, etc.

Technical comparisons of visual display terminal- and television-application of cathode ray tubes. Compared with television (TV) sets, 'modern' VDTs tend to employ higher refresh rates (commonly 70 Hz or higher compared to 50/60 Hz), in order to avoid flicker, especially at high luminances.

Higher refresh rates also require higher horizontal sweep frequencies (from TVs 15 kHz to 25 kHz or higher), and thus faster changes in the magnetic field strength of the deflecting coils. This latter increase is however offset to some degree by the use of a lower acceleration potential (in monochromatic VDTs).

Higher sweep frequencies as well as a demand for higher resolution also require higher modulation frequencies and thus higher signal bandwidths. (Restrictions to the TV/radio frequency bandwidth would seriously interfere with pixel size - causing it to spread horizontally and interfere with legibility.)

The phosphors used in VDTs must be determined according to colour, persistence, etc. CRT phosphors vary considerably in persistence time. Phosphors used for display purposes normally have persistence times of around 100 μsec or longer. These persistence values may vary considerably however between different investigations.

A brief review is found in Baldauf (1985).

5.2.2 Electromagnetic radiation and fields from visual display terminals

VDTs based on the cathode ray tube are a source of several distinct types
of electromagnetic radiations. Such emissions are characterized by a number
of interdependent parameters. Some of these parameters relate to the 'type'
of radiation: frequency, wavelength or photon energy. Others refer to the
'amount' of radiation: irradiance/power density or illuminance. The range of
the electromagnetic spectrum in term of frequency (or related parameters) is
given in Table 1.

The electromagnetic field has both an electric (E) and a magnetic (B or H)
component, and the relations between them are rather complex. For practical
reasons, the field is separated in a 'near-field' (less than 1 wavelength from
the source) and a 'far-field'. At the operator's distance from the VDT, the
near-field is of interest when discussing radiofrequencies and very low or
extremely low frequencies. In this near-field, the electric and magnetic
fields must be characterized separately, and, e.g., occupational standards are
set separately for these two components.

A further complication is due to the fact that most measurements are
related to the emission from the VDT, while standards are set at exposure to
the person. For practical reasons, this can be met for many radiation
categories by measuring emission at a relevant distance from the VDT. Thus,
measurements are overestimating exposure by measuring levels closer to the
screen. For a low-frequency electric field, this simple approach is not
appropriate. It will be discussed further on page 38 for extremely low
frequency fields, and on pages 44-45 for electrostatic fields.

Table 1.   Electromagnetic emissions from VDTs

Denotation[a]	Range[a]	VDTs as a potential source[b]	Emission, upper limit[c]	Standards[d]	Number of VDTs examined[e]
Ionizing radiation[f]					
X-ray radiation	more than 1.2 keV	yes	ND[g] (probably much less than 0.1 mSv/yr)[g]	5-10 mSv/yr	more than 3000
Ionizing UV	12 eV-1.2 keV	no[h]			
Optical radiation[f]					
UV_{BC} (actinic)	200-315 nm	no	10 $\mu W/m^2$ (=0.3 J/m^2, 8h)	30 J/m^2, 24h	more than 200
UV_A	315-400 nm	yes[i]	0.1 W/m^2	10 W/m^2	appr. 500
Light	400-700 nm	yes	2.5 W/m^2 127 cd/m^2	10 000cd/m^2	appr. 500 136
Near IR	700-1050 nm	yes[i]	0.05 W/m^2	100 W/m^2	more than 200
Far IR	1050 nm-1 mm	yes[k]	4 W/m^{2}[k]		
Hertzian radiation and fields[l]					
Microwaves (UHF, SHF, EHF)	300 MHz- 300 GHz	no	ND[m]	10-100 W/m^2	more than 300
HF, VHF					
E-Field	3 MHz-300 MHz	yes	0.5 V/m	100 V/m[n]	more than 300
H-Field		yes	0.0002 A/m	0.2 A/m[n]	3
VLF, MF, LF					
E-field	3 kHz-3 MHz	yes	150 V/m	600 V/m[n]	appr. 400
H-Field		yes	0.1 A/m	1.6 A/m[n]	47
ELF					
E-field	0-3 kHz	yes	65 V/m[o]	2-10 kV/m[p]	5
H-field		yes	0.2 A/m	-	4
Electrostatic fields					
Electro- static	0 Hz	yes[q]	15 kV/m[r]	20-60 kV/m[s]	appr. 500

UV = ultraviolet; IR = infrared; HF = high frequency; UHF = ultra high frequency; SHF = super high frequency; EHF = extra high frequency; VHF = very high frequency; VLF = very low frequency; MF = medium frequency; LF = low frequency; ELF = extremely low frequency.

Notes for Table 1:

<u>a</u> Range is given in energy (eV) for ionizing radiation, in wavelength (m) for optical radiation, and in frequency (Hz) for 'Hertzian' radiation and fields. The denotations and ranges do differ between different authors. The terms "Hertzian" is used here, instead of radiofrequency fields, which is also used, but which does not always include ELF fields. For frequencies below 300 MHz, the field is separated into an electric (E) and a magnetic (H) component.

<u>b</u> This refers to knowledge of processes within the VDT that may give rise to emissions.

<u>c</u> Highest level recorded, which is attributed to the VDT. Note that spurious readings, due to instrument inadequacies or errors, have been reported (see further text). ND = not detected.

<u>d</u> Approximate, refer to standards, guidelines or recommendations as set in several countries. For detailed information, see text. Note also that standards may not apply to the whole region. Data here are introduced for a rough comparison only.

<u>e</u> In reviewed studies.

<u>f</u> Includes measurements made 'close' to the screen.

<u>g</u> See pp. 33-34 for discussion on measurements deviating from these conclusions - made under extreme test conditions. The probable emission is derived from laboratory measurements on some VDTs (see further below).

<u>h</u> Ionizing radiation with photon energies less than 5 keV, (vacuum UV), is of no practical interest, since these photons do not penetrate air.

<u>i</u> Depends on the phosphor.

<u>k</u> Heat emission occurs, due to surface temperature below $32^{\circ}C$ (Cox, 1984).

$\underline{l}$ Normally measured at 30 cm distance.

$\underline{m}$ Spurious readings have been reported, see text.

$\underline{n}$ USSR standards generally permit higher magnetic fields, but lower electric fields.

$\underline{o}$ Does not refer to unperturbed fields. (In such case, the level would probably be about 10 V/m.)

$\underline{p}$ At power frequency 50/60 Hz.

$\underline{q}$ Depending on surface conductivity of the screen.

$\underline{r}$ Does not refer to unperturbed fields. (The range of the electrostatic fields in the operator situation from 400 VDT work stations was 0–15 kV/m, see text.)

$\underline{s}$ USSR limits.

Most measurements made are averaged over time (rms, during the whole pertinent cycle) and over space (for at least a substantial part of the screen). This is possibly inappropriate in some specific situations, two of which have been given some attention:

- Nonsinusoidal magnetic fields, where the change in time of the magnetic field may be of interest; and

- Light, where the individual pixels radiate most energy during a limited time of each cycle.

5.2.2.1 <u>Potential electromagnetic radiations and fields</u>. A visual display terminal based on the CRT is a potential source of several distinct electromagnetic spectral bands. The actual intensity of each band, frequencies, etc., depend on the detailed technical design of the terminal, shielding, as well as other factors.

Band 1. <u>X-ray radiation</u> arises within the CRT tube when the accelerated electrons are quickly slowed down by the screen material. The energies of these photons are limited by the acceleration potential.

Band 2. <u>Optical radiations</u> are purposely derived by the phosphor material in the screen, when interacting with the electrons. The overall (time average) emission levels are discussed in this section, while details of light emissions are discussed under display characteristics. Adjacent to the visible spectrum, some emission of near ultraviolet and near infrared may occur.

Band 3. <u>High frequency radio fields</u> do appear, apparently related to the frequency of pixel formation and the intensity modulations of the incident electron beam towards the screen, regulating the intensity of the dots on the screeen. This frequency is then related to the frequency of the information signal system. (Such signals are of interest in attempts to 'spy' on a VDT.)

Band 4. <u>Low frequency radio fields</u> emanate from the horizontal deflection system (flyback transformer, connecting wires and the screen), with a purposedly created magnetic field.

Band 5. Extremely low frequency fields (ELF) arise around the refresh rate
        (vertical sweep frequency), and apparently depend on both the
        vertical deflection system (producing a purposeful magnetic field)
        and, possibly also, on modulations of the electrostatic field
        (positive electrostatic charge modulated by the intermittent negative
        electron beam).

Band 6. Electrostatic fields frequently appear, related to the acceleration
        potential of the CRT and the conductivity of the screen surface.

   Radiations whose time dependence cannot be described by a simple
sinusoidal function (of a certain frequency) give rise to 'harmonics' of
higher frequencies and lower amplitudes. Thus, the bands 3 to 5 (above) each
include a fundamental frequency and several harmonics of higher frequencies
(most of the energy normally being confined to frequencies within 10 times the
fundamental frequency).

   Most regions are heavily dependent on the mode of operation of the VDT.
This has been explicitly shown for bands 3 and 5 (and is self-evident for band
2). By special measures (blinking cursor, interlace, etc.), subharmonics can
appear - as shown for the electric component of band 5). (See also pp. 22-25
for a brief description of VDT/CRT technical design.)

   Data on sound emission is presented on pages 47-48.

5.2.2.2 Ionizing radiation. Considerable attention has been given to
reported cases of miscarriages, skin rashes and cataracts among VDT-
operators. Since VDTs are potential sources of X-rays, possible causes of
these effects, a discussion of performed measurements on X-ray emissions from
VDTs is appropriate.

   The potential source of X-rays within a VDT is the cathode ray tube, and
specifically the inside of the fluorescent viewing screen. The energy of the
photons is limited by the high voltage used to accelerate electrons, to some
10 - 25 keV (soft X-rays). Due to their limited energies, these X-ray
emissions are effectively absorbed by the glass screen (Repacholi, 1985; Zuk
et al., 1983).

X-ray measurements performed on VDTs in field conditions. Some 3000 terminals have been measured for possible X-ray emission, in for example, Austria, Canada, Italy, Sweden, the United Kingdom and the USA (Bureau of Radiological Health, 1981; Cox, 1984; Moss et al., 1977; Paulsson et al., 1984; Phillips, 1981; Terrana et al., 1982; Weiss & Petersen, 1979; Wolbarscht et al., 1980; Zuk et al., 1983). Several models and units were tested in more than one investigation. Most units were tested at 5 cm or less from the screen under normal operating conditions (often with maximum brightness and full screen). No measurements in field conditions have detected any X-ray emission from VDTs (i.e. being detectable above the background of some 0.1-0.2 μSv/h). A detailed summary of most of these measurements is found in Zuk et al. (1983).[1]

Bell Canada tested 925 units and reported levels in the range up to 0.0-2.0 μGy/h. However, the test results as presented contained some anomalies, such as an apparent dependency on the measuring instrument. The Radiation Protection Bureau in Canada retested several of the tested units and failed to find any emission. The Bureau found the Bell Canada measurements to be erroneous (Zuk et al., 1983).

X-ray measurements performed on VDTs under laboratory conditions. Radiation testing was performed on 125 VDTs by the US Bureau of Radiological Health (1981), which used also 'Phase III' test conditions (these test specifications include maximum voltage and worst-case component or circuit fault still compatible with a legible screen) in order to find the theoretical X-ray emission maximum. Eleven of the 125 units did under these artificial test conditions emit measurable levels; three at less than 4.4 μGy/h and eight at 4.4-17.6 μGy/h.

Efforts have been made to detect the actual X-ray emission from VDTs by various methods. In a detection chamber (shielded from background), 52 units were examined without any emission being found. The limit of detection was reported to be 10^{-11} Gy/h (Pomroy & Noel, 1984). There was no change in the

---

1 For electromagnetic radiation, the absorbed dose (Gy) and the dose equivalent (Sv) are numerically the same. Furthermore, 1 rad = 0.01 Gy, 1 rem = 0.01 Sv. 1 R (röntgen) = 2.58 x 10^{-4} Ckg^{-1} (ionization in air).

background measurements when the VDT was switched on. Similar findings were reported by Paulsson and coworkers (1984) and Phillips (1981). By using a NaI (Tl) scintillation detector and pulse height analyser, an emission of 25 nGy/h was detected from a VDT. Emission bands appeared at 5, 15 and 30 keV. The operating conditions were normal, with full screen. The same VDT gave off an additional 25 nGy/h at 20 keV under fault conditions (Wolbarscht et al., 1980).

Compliance with emission standards. In many countries, product emission standards for CRTs (applicable to VDTs) are set at 0.5 mR/h. (Full-time exposure to this would be equivalent of 7 mSv/yr.) It is apparent that practically all VDTs tested (more than 99%) comply with these emission standards. Those failing to do so (only found during Phase III test conditions, see above), were removed from or denied access to the USA market. [These product standards are considered to be more than sufficient for the protection of the skin, the fetus and the eyes. Some discussion may be in order for breast and thyroid gland doses, according to Hirning and Aitken, (1982).]

The national standard for the population at large (not radiation workers) in, for example Sweden, is 5 mSv/year. Extensive testing of VDTs under operating conditions has failed to detect any VDT with X-ray emissions giving dose equivalents in excess of these standards.[1] In general, no ionizing radiation was detected unless elaborate detection procedures were used to eliminate the background influence. [In one study by Paulsson et al. (1984), a 'decrease' in the background levels was actually noted close to the screen, due to some shielding of the background by the VDT.]

5.2.2.3 Optical radiation. The range of wavelengths (100 nm to 1 mm) constituting 'optical radiation' comprises non-ionizing ultraviolet (UV), light and infrared (IR) radiations.

---

1 Theoretically, the annual maximum permissible dose to a member of the public could be exceeded for operators sitting very close to one of the eight 'non-compliance' VDT models during the phase III test conditions. However, any reasonable assumptions as to viewing distances, attenuation, shielding, normal technical working conditions of the VDT, etc., result in a dose equivalent from VDTs far below these standards.

The UV region of 200-315 nm is termed 'actinic' UV (comprises UV-B/mid-UV/erythemal UV and UV-C/far-UV/germicidal UV. UV-C also includes some 'vacuum' UV, which does not penetrate air). Actinic UV is associated with most biological effects ascribed to UV radiation (Hughes, 1982a; WHO, 1979).

IR radiation is separated into near infrared (wavelengths 700-1050 nm) and far infrared.

The spectral emission curves of CRT phosphors show a varied distribution throughout the 300 to 800 nm band (light and UV and IR bands adjacent to the visible region).

Measurements of UV radiation. Actinic UV (UV-B and UV-C) from VDTs are generally not detectable (Cox, 1984; Paulsson et al., 1984; Wolbarscht et al., 1980). In a few instances, detectable levels [1 μW/m^2 (0.5 m)] (Wolbarscht et al., 1980), and 10 μW/m^2 (close) (Paulsson et al., 1984) have been detected. These levels were below the limit of detection in most investigations.

Measurements in the near UV region will depend on the phosphor used. In general, UV emissions occur with blue-green phosphors, but not with yellow-orange ones (Walsh & Facey, 1983). In the majority (85%) of these measurements, no UV-A radiation was detectable, with levels in those detectable normally around 0.001 W/m^2 (close) (Bureau of Radiological Health, 1981; Cox, 1984; Moss et al., 1977; Murray et al., 1981a; Murray et al., 1981b; Paulsson et al., 1984; Phillips, 1981; Weiss, 1983; Weiss & Petersen, 1979; Wolbarscht et al., 1980). The maximum level detected was 0.12 W/m^2 (close) (Cox, 1984).

In an investigation by Knave and coworkers (1985a), the level of ambient UV-A radiation was about 0.04 W/m^2 for VDT-operators, and 0.13 W/m^2 for non-VDT operators. In both situations the detector was aimed towards the ceiling. The authors interpreted this by the major UV-A sources being windows and fluorescent lights, and since VDT-operators worked in darker rooms, exposure would decrease due to work with VDTs.

<u>Measurements of visible radiation</u>. The irradiance of light from the VDTs
tested varied between less than 0.1 W/m^2 and 2.5 W/m^2, and did also show
an (expected) distance variation (Bureau of Radiological Health, 1981; Cox,
1984; Murray et al., 1981b; Weiss, 1983; Wolbarscht et al., 1980). The
radiance was 0.1 W/m^2,sr (sr=sterradian or spare angle) in one investigation
by Wolbarscht et al. (1980), in reasonable concordance with the luminance
levels of 3.4 - 127 cd/m^2 found by Murray et al. (1981b). (Note that the
radiance and luminance values are not distance dependent.)

The time variation of the emission may however be considerable for 'fast'
phosphors. For a P$_{31}$ phosphor, a decay time of 11 us was noted, which
suggests a top luminance of about 65 000 cd/m^2 (Nylén & Bergqvist, 1986).
However, the American Conference of Governmental Industrial Hygienists (ACGIH,
1983) TLV guideline levels (spectrally weighted), are still considerably
higher than the emission levels of these phosphors.

<u>Measurements of infrared radiation</u>. The highest near IR measurement was
0.05 W/m^2 (close), while no far infrared was detected apart from heat
emission (equivalent of less than 32°C) according to Cox (1984).

<u>Compliance with standards</u>. Comparison with some available standards
(Swedish, ACGIH) reveals that the noted highest emissions from VDTs are about
two orders of magnitude below these standards.

A spectral analysis was made on two VDTs (Paulsson et al., 1984) and the
retinal thermal injury weighted radiation was found to be 0.12 and 0.29
W/m^2,sr, respectively, to be compared with the ACGIH TLV standard of 10^2
W/m^2,sr [long-term exposure (ACGIH, 1983)].

5.2.2.4 <u>Hertzian[1] radiation and fields</u>. In this section, electromagnetic
radiation frequencies below 300 GHz are discussed. This frequency range is
used extensively by a large number of ubiquitous technical appliances [radio,
TV, microwave ovens, radar etc., see the World Health Organization publication
(1981)] and also includes fields inadvertently caused by the common net

---

1 The name 'Hertzian' implies frequencies below 300 GHz. In many countries,
the term radiofrequency would be synonymous.

frequency 50 Hz (60 Hz in Canada or USA). The frequency range is separated
below into microwave, high radio frequencies (VHF, HF), low radio frequencies
(MF, LF, VLF) and extremely low frequencies (ELF) (see Table 1 for demarcation
limits).

A comprehensive review of measurement techniques and results by Guy (1984)
is available. Further tabulations of the data presented here are found in
Bergqvist (1984) and Zuk and coworkers (1983).

Measurements of microwave radiation from VDTs. Cox (1984) measured fields
in the region 300 MHz - 18 GHz around more than 200 VDTs. For one VDT, a
measure of 5 W/m^2 was recorded, the rest were below 1 W/m^2. Cox (1984)
retested some of these tested VDTs with other measuring instruments, and did
get considerably lower measurements - which he attributed to some recording
instruments being sensitive also to other frequency ranges.

Phillips (1981) failed to detect any microwave radiation on 114 VDTs
(limit of detection was 0.5 W/m^2 with one instrument, and 0.1 W/m^2 with
another). Some low and isolated readings were also recorded from about 1.4
GHz, but they were interpreted as being "associated with the computer and not
the display terminal in the same room" (Weiss & Petersen, 1979).

The absence of microwave generating circuits, and of detectable and
verified measurements of microwave emissions from VDTs, are the basis for the
conclusion that VDTs are not sources of microwave emissions.

Measurements of high radio frequency (VHF, HF) fields around VDTs. In
some studies, strong electric and magnetic field strengths (of the order of
10^3 V/m and 1 A/m, respectively) were measured (Murray et al., 1981a;
Stuchly et al., 1983a). These measurement results were apparently due to a
capacitive coupling between the Narda meter and the fly-back transformer.
Other instruments, when used on the same VDTs, have not confirmed these high
readings (Bureau of Radiological Health, 1981; Stuchly et al., 1983a; Zuk et
al., 1983).

Using more sensitive instruments, however, consistent measurements have
been obtained in the MHz region. These fields appear very localized, and thus

vary considerably with distance, with the position of the measuring instrument around the VDT and with the activity of the VDT. Typical field strength readings vary between less than 1 mV/m at 1 m distance to 0.5 V/m 'at surface' (E-field) and probably between 0.1 and 200 μA/m (H field, 5-30 cm distance). The frequency range used by these emanations is 1 to 200 MHz, with most activities concentrated around about 3 - 30 MHz (Bureau of Radiological Health, 1981; Cox, 1984; Harvey, 1984; Moss et al., 1977; Terrana et al., 1982; Weiss & Petersen, 1979; Wolbarscht et al., 1980).

Measurements of low radio frequency (MF, LF, VLF) fields around VDTs. Electromagnetic fields around VDTs in the frequency range 10 kHz - 1 MHz have consistently been detected in a number of investigations. This frequency range corresponds to the horizontal sweep frequency (normally 15 - 50 kHz) and its major harmonics (i.e. multiples of this fundamental frequency). In some investigations, at least 95% of the total field strength (all radio frequencies) was accounted for by the fundamental frequency and its five next harmonics, corresponding to the range of some 15 to 125 kHz. This appeared true of both the E- and the H-field strength (Bureau of Radiological Health, 1981). Other measurements indicate a wider spread of at least the magnetic field frequencies (Paulsson et al., 1984).

The results show an E-field strength of between 0.3 and 150 V/m and an H-field of some 0.05 A/m (at approximately 30 cm distance) (Bureau of Radiological Health, 1981; Cox, 1984; Paulsson et al., 1984; Terrana et al., 1982; Weiss, 1983; Weiss & Petersen, 1979; Wolbarscht et al., 1980; Zuk et al., 1983).

Measurements of extremely low frequency electric and magnetic fields (ELF) around VDTs. Few measurements have been made in this region. As suggested by these results, the electric and magnetic fields strength in this region are comparable to those of the low radio frequency (kHz) region (above); some 50 V/m (E-field) and 0.1 - 0.2 A/m (H-field) (Harvey, 1984; Stuchly et al., 1983a). It should be noted that the E-field measured by Harvey (1984) is not an unperturbed field - some theoretical evaluations suggest that these fields should be divided by a factor of 10 to arrive at the unperturbed field.

The real time appearance and the distance dependence of the magnetic
fields. The magnetic fields are due to the requirements for electron beam
deflection, and are thus related to the maximum deflection angle of the beam
and to the scanning (horizontal sweep) and the refresh (vertical sweep)
rates. The principal appearances of these fields are shown in Figure 2. The
real time appearances of the total magnetic fields are fairly complex, since
they are formed by several constituent fields of varied location and frequency
(Paulsson et al., 1984). Descriptions of these fields in terms of their
Fourier transforms are discussed by Guy (1984).

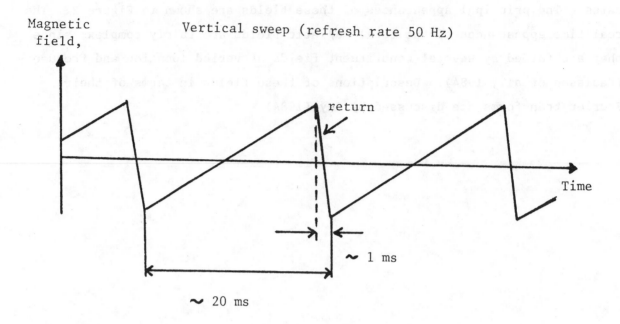

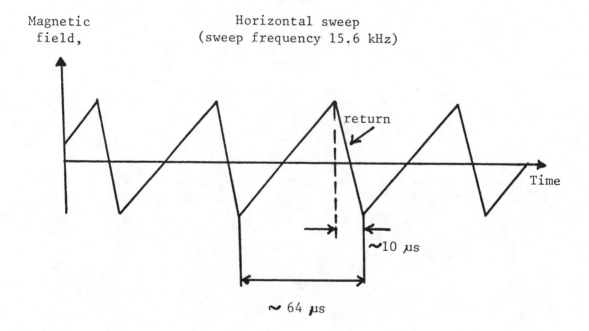

Fig. 2: Principal real time appearance of pulsed magnetic fields used for horizontal and vertical deflections of the electron beam. (The real appearance of these fields can be quite complex.)

With a B-field strength (kHz region at 30 cm) of 0.07 μT (H=0.06 A/m), the time derivative of the field (dB/dt) will be of the order of 10 mT/s during the 'return time' (based on the appearance in Figure 2). In the ELF region, a typical value for dB/dt (from the vertical sweep) is about 0.5 mT/s (30 cm distance).

The range of dB/dt (all frequencies 50 Hz - 300 kHz) has been measured by Paulsson and coworkers (1984) for a number of VDTs: 13.5 mT/s (0.3 m, 43 VDTs), 2.3 mT/s (0.7 m, 7 VDTs) and 0.8 mT/s (1 m, 28 VDTs). The range at 0.3 m distance was 1 to 43 mT/s.

A summary of further measurements have been presented by Paulsson (1986). Levels of dB/dt at 30 cm distance varied between 7 and 580 mT/s. Modern screens tended to have higher dB/dt-levels than older screens, primarily due to a higher sweep frequencies - but examples of low dB/dt levels for modern screens with high sweep frequencies were also noted.

The E- and H-fields (kHz region) were found to be radially directed from the VDT screen (Bureau of Radiological Health, 1981). According to Paulsson and coworkers (1984), the total (all frequencies) H-field had a varied direction, with sizeable components along all three coordinates.

The electromagnetic fields from the VDT decrease quickly with increasing distance. The degree by which these fields appear to decrease varies however between VDT models and also between investigations (possibly influenced by varying instrumental sensitivity at varying distances). Paulsson and coworkers (1984) showed that the H-field strength (50 Hz-300 kHz) decreased at approximately r^{-3} with distance, although considerable variations from this were found for many individual models.

Compliance of VDT emissions with existing standards. In Sweden, proposed occupational standards for radio frequency fields encompass the frequency region 3 MHz - 300 GHz. Within this region, field strengths in the band 3 MHz - 30 MHz should not exceed 140 V/m (E-field) and 0.4 A/m (H-field), while the maximum permissible field strengths in the band 30 MHz - 300 MHz are 60 V/m and 0.16 A/m respectively (NBOSH, 1985a). These limits are in general agreement with those of the National Standards Institute in the USA and ACGIH and international recommendations of the International Radiation Protection Association (IRPA). The high radio frequency field strengths measured around VDTs are orders of magnitude below these standards.

In the 10 kHz to 3 MHz region, the ACGIH has adopted a threshold limit value (TLV) of 600 V/m (E-field) and 1.6 A/m (H-field). These values are somewhat higher than those of the IRPA, the latter however being confined to above 100 kHz, or, for the E-field, the USSR limits, although these are valid only for frequencies of 60 KHz and higher (ACGIH, 1983; USSR, 1984; WHO, 1981). The levels measured from VDTs in this region are considerably below these occupational standards.

No standards exist for part of the low radio frequency and the VLF/ELF regions. Some guidelines for exposure limits for 50/60 Hz E-fields have been given, however. These limits are generally found in the 1-10 kV/m range (USSR, 1984; WHO, 1984), i.e. far above measured levels at VDTs.

Comparison with other exposures. Evaluation of emissions in these regions are made also from other points - especially for the magnetic fields. Comparison with other exposures in industry or households shows that the levels found at VDTs are orders of magnitude lower than several other exposure situations, when comparison is made according to the amplitude (B). Comparisons made according to dB/dt are more difficult, since measurements are seldom given for this parameter. Available data do however indicate that there are several exposure situations where the exposure as dB/dt is considerably above those found around VDTs. (See some data in Paulsson et al., 1984.)

A major problem is that there are no data to determine what parameter (B, dB/dt or other) should be used for comparison. This is due to the lack of any established or clearly indicated effects for relevant domains in frequency and amplitude - and thus to what mechanisms may be involved. In a recent study by Juutilainen & Saali (1986), some effects of ELF and VLF magnetic fields on chick embryogenesis were indicated. The authors concluded that "the effect (dH/dt) suggests that the interaction mechanism is other than induction of electric currents by the magnetic field". In the following paragraphs, discussed mechanisms are considered.

Specific absorption rates. Thermal mechanisms are thought to be responsible for many of the effects on biological systems seen after exposure to microwave and radiofrequency radiation (WHO, 1981). The relative energy absorption of radiofrequency fields decreases with decreasing frequencies [see the discussion on specific absorption rates (SAR) by Guy (1980)]. Thus, the E-and H-field strengths recorded in the low radio frequency and very low frequency regions are not expected to cause any effect (which depends on thermal mechanisms). Calculations for energy deposition from typical fields have been made, and are totally insignificant compared to metabolic heat (Stuchly et al., 1983b).

Resonance frequencies (allowing for non-thermal effects) have been under considerable discussion lately. No such resonance phenomena have, so far been shown for frequencies and intensities of interest when discussing VDTs.

Induced currents. The rate of change of the magnetic field (dB/dt) is physically coupled to an induced current in the medium. This current is determined also by the size of the structure (in the body) used for calculations. There are however no data to indicate what structure to use for the possibility of fetal malformation. The currents induced by the sweep frequency's dB/dt (15-50 kHz) have been calculated as 0.1-10 mAs/m^2 in peripheral parts of the body, based on a current path around the body. Currents in smaller structures, such as cell structures, will be correspondingly lower. The body's own current range from 1-1000 mAs/m^2, but are limited to frequencies below 1 kHz. Some electrical handtools will cause similar current in the frequency range 1-10 kHz (Paulsson et al., 1984).

Guy (1984) evaluated the data from his own and others' measurements of VDT electromagnetic fields. He discussed the experiments of Delgado and coworkers (1982) on the effects of bone growth stimulations by magnetic fields. In his recommendations, Guy states that "Until this validity issue is resolved, critics will use the results of the above works to argue that the level of emissions from VDTs is not safe." In respect to the electric fields he states: "It certainly is desirable to shield the cover of the VDT. Since such shielding is relatively inexpensive the benefit-to-cost ratio is large. Such shielding is generally present in newer models of VDTs to satisfy FCC requirements for reducing electromagnetic interference." The apparent ambiguity in his writing concerning shielding has lead to debate on the issue. In a later foreword to his report, Guy added "In my report, I acknowledge that the electric-field measurements of a particular older model display as well as the unverified reports (both Soviet and Delgado) of biological effects from lower level fields may be used by some to argue that VDTs are not safe. In that context, I find that the shielding as now required by the FCC in newer displays is desirable since it is reassuring to those concerned. I do not feel, however, that unshielded VDT emission levels represent a potential health hazard. I remain convinced based on the evidence that VDTs are safe to use." A further discussion on possible biological effects of low frequency magnetic fields may be found in the section on adverse pregnancy outcomes (pp. 143-145)

5.2.2.5 Electrostatic fields. Screens of CRT design frequently attain an electrostatic charge when in operation. No explanation of the cause of these charges and fields has been published, but they can readily be assumed to be dependent on the following factors: first, the Post Acceleration Potential (PAP) commonly used in CRT devices to accelerate the electrons towards the screen. The PAP is applied to the metal-coated inside of the screen, and may amount to 20 kV or more (Grivet, 1972). Secondly, the screen itself should ideally serve as a shield for the field associated with this potential charge, but this shielding may be imperfect, supposedly due to the limited conductance of the screen itself. Thirdly, accumulation of charged particles on the screen surface will decrease the resultant field. Fourthly, the relative humidity will affect the recorded electrostatic field, since it will affect the conductance of the screen material.

In a study by Bergqvist and coworkers (1986), the electrostatic field from a VDT was recorded during a period of time after switching on and then off. The field strength peaked immediately after switching on, and then gradually decreased to a semi-steady level. When the VDT was switched off, a negative field strength was recorded, which gradually decreased.

Measurements of electrostatic fields from VDTs. A few reports on measurements of electrostatic fields associated with this charge have been published. The results indicate fairly large variations in the measured electrostatic field from different VDTs, with means in different studies between 8 and 75 kV/m under varying measurement conditions (Cato Olsen, 1981; Harvey, 1984, Knave et al. 1985b, Paulsson et al., 1984). When comparing these data, the causes of the varying values must be considered.

Differences according to measuring procedures. In the investigations by Cato Olsen (1981) and Knave et al. (1985b), both used the same procedures; the placement of a field mill in a central position in front of the screen. The mill was grounded and the field strength was noted. Both Harvey (1984) and Paulsson and coworkers (1984) used a measuring procedure supplemented by placing a large earthed metal plate adjacent to the field mill, with the field mill sensor in a hole made in the plate. The latter procedure is less vulnerable to distortions of the measured field. The introduction of the large grounded plate, however, also changes the field geometry considerably, causing a substantial decrease in the field strength, and direct comparisons between the results of the two procedures are not possible.

Differences according to distance. Paulsson and coworkers (1984) found that the electrostatic field decreased as r^{-1} 'close' to the screen, and as r^{-3} at 'larger' distances from the screen.

By attempting to compensate for these differences, the results of the mean of the four studies cited above was in the 4 to 12 kV/m range - at 30 cm distance.

The approximate potential on the VDT screen. In attempting to eliminate the influence of the measurement geometry, the potential on the screen was estimated, using methods by Harvey (1984): the average screen potentials were then 1.5 kV (Cato Olsen, 1981), 2.0 kV (Harvey, 1984), 4.4 kV (Paulsson et al., 1984) and 5.0 kV (Knave et al., 1985b). These differences may be due to different makes being examined. In Knave et al. (1985b), a number of VDTs from seven different makes were examined. Two makes exhibited almost no field, one make had a fairly small field, and four makes had a large field. Similar patterns were also seen in other investigations (Cato Olsen, 1981; Paulsson et al., 1984).

The electrostatic potential of the operator. Numerous data exist on the electrostatic potential of human beings. The potentials of VDT-operators have been measured based on data from Cato Olsen (1981), by the same methods that were used to measure the screen potential described above. Of 78 measurements (on 16 individuals), 47% had a negative potential between - 2.2 and -0.2 kV (mean ca -0.9 kV), 28% had a potential close to zero (between -0.2 kV and + 0.2 kV), while 22% had a positive potential between +0.2 kV and +2.2 kV (mean ca +1.1 kV). Two persons (3%) had a positive potential of +3.8 to +4.2 kV. The overall mean potential was -0.6 kV.

Similar calculations on measurements referred to in Knave et al. (1985b) indicate that the average potential of operators were more positive (mean - 5 V) than were controls (mean -40 V). This has been attributed to a number of VDT operators working at grounded metal keyboards.

It should be noted that the measurements by Cato Olsen (1981) were made in an office with substantial 'electrostatic' annoyance, while those of Knave and coworkers (1985b) were made in a random ('normal') selection of offices. In an experimental study, the electrostatic potential of the operator was independent of the electrostatic field from the VDT (Bergqvist et al., 1986).

The electrostatic field between the VDT and the operator. A rough estimate of the electrostatic field between the operator and the screen can be derived from the formula:

$$E = (V_{screen} - V_{operator})/r$$

(E = electrostatic field strength, V = Potential, r = distance between the screen and the operator.)

In the investigation by Cato Olsen (1981), the field between the 'average' VDT and the 'average' person would then be about 3.5 kV/m. In Knave and coworkers (1985b), the calculated fields for each workstation varied between 0 and 15 kV/m.

In a recent paper, Cato Olsen (1986) discusses the relative importance of the VDT and the operator potentials. In situations where static electricity is a problem, model measurements showed that the operator potential was the dominating factor for particle deposition.

5.2.2.6 <u>Sound and noise from visual display terminals</u>. Some VDTs are potential sources of several sonic frequencies, in both the audible and the ultrasound range. This noise may conceivably have some bearing on certain aspects of physiological and psychological discomfort.

<u>Measurements of sound and noise</u>. The levels of acoustic radiation emanating from VDTs have been measured by the US Bureau of Radiological Health (1981) and were found to fall within the frequency range 6.3 kHz - 40 kHz. The dominant frequencies from the 25 tested VDTs were between 16 kHz to 40 kHz, related to the horizontal sweep frequency. The noise supposedly originated in the flyback transformer core. However, the frequency used in this transformer is often too high for the audible range, especially of middle aged people. It is possible that secondary noise sources (with half the frequency of the transformer) may exist within the VDT units.

The sound pressure levels (SPL) at about 50 cm from the VDT in the direction of maximum emission were within the 30 to 68 dB range (mean 51 dB). In the 16 - 20 kHz range, the maximum registered level was 61 dB (mean 53 db) (Bureau of Radiological Health, 1981). Similar data have also been presented by Paulsson (1986).

The mean SPL of 14 of these VDTs was 52 dB at the horizontal sweep frequency with a lower SPL (mean 44 dB) at the double frequency. For five VDTs, the opposite was true: mean 47 dB at sweep frequency, 49 dB (mean) at the double frequency. For all these VDTs, the sweep frequencies were 20 kHz or lower, while the double frequencies were above 20 kHz. One VDT had a higher SPL (51 dB) at half the sweep frequency than at the sweep frequency (44 dB at ca 35 kHz) (Bureau of Radiological Health, 1981).

<u>Compliance with standards</u>. Swedish occupational standards limit the sound pressure level at 20 kHz and above to between 105 and 115 dB (relative to 20 μPa) (NBOSH, 1978). At 8 - 20 kHz, the level is 80 dB. For 'single tones' (conceivably the case here), the corresponding limit is 70 dB (NBOSH, 1976). Available information suggests that VDTs comply with present standards as to dangerous noise levels in the 6 kHz range to 40 KHz range.

A correlation between complaints of noise from VDTs and emotional or mood complaints was noted by Stammerjohn (1981). It has been suggested that high frequency noise might be a stress factor, and that noise from VDTs may cause 'sensory overload' (Wolf S. personal communication). So far, these suggestions have not been substantiated.

5.2.3 Display characteristics and workroom lighting

The information received by the operator is derived from that of the screen, subject to the legibility of the screen characters. A number of parameters are relevant to a discussion of discomfort or health effects (e.g. asthenopia) and job performance. These parameters have been divided into three groups, relating to the oscillation, the structure and the luminance of the presented symbols and the screen. Workroom illumination parameters are included in this section, since they are closely interrelated with the display parameters in defining, for example, screen contrast.

Reading performance is discussed as an indication of adverse display presentation only — the rationale being that adverse reading performance will be related to eye discomfort, and as a stress factor, etc. (For further discussions, see Bouma, 1982; Engel, 1982; National Research Council, 1983; Radl, 1982; Timmers, 1982).

5.2.3.1 Time-dependent variables of screen luminants

Pixel illumination rates. As decribed on pp. 23-25, the electron beam in a CRT device sweeps across the pixels, producing an illuminated dot or a line segment.

A typical vertical sweep time of 19 ms (and a return time of 1 ms) corresponds to a refresh rate (repetition of each 'pixel' irradiation) of 50 Hz. Refresh rates between 56 and 77 Hz (typically 60 Hz[1]) were noted by the US Bureau of Radiological Health (1981) and between 48 and 81 Hz (typically 50 Hz[1]) by the Swedish SSI [National Institute of Radiation Protection (Paulsson et al., 1984).]

---

1 Net frequency in the USA is 60 Hz, as opposed to the European one of 50 Hz.

The horizontal sweep frequencies did vary considerable in the Bureau of Radiological Health investigation (1981), between 2 and 35 kHz (typically 15 - 20 kHz), and between 15 and 53 kHz (typically 15 - 25 kHz) in the Swedish investigation (Paulsson et al., 1984). The return times varied between 2.8 and 10 us (mean ca 6 us).

A horizontal sweep time of 54 us (line frequency 15.6 kHz) corresponds to some 230 - 300 lines/frame (with some time allowed for return time etc.). With a character matrix of 7x9 'pixels' and 80 characters/line, the passage time is about 0.1 μs/'pixel'. The information frequency needed for beam modulation (gate potential, Fig. 1) is then of the order of 10 MHz and higher.

Oscillation of pixel lumination. The real time appearance of the 'pixel' luminance is shown in Fig. 3, both for a fast and a slow phosphor. Phosphor decay times (from 100% to 10% of maximum luminance) vary considerably with the phosphor, and they also vary considerably between different investigations.

The decay time for different cathode ray phosphors varies between extremely fast (P_{16} - used in certain radar installations - 0.16 μs) to extremely slow (P_{34} - 100 sec). Typical decay times for phosphors used in VDT applications are about 60 us (P_4), 24 ms (P_{22G}), 30 μs (P_{31}) and 1.2 ms (P_{43}) (Westinghouse, 1972). (For a P_{22G} phosphor, decay times of 6 ms (data from IBM Corp) to 60 μs (data from Clinton Corp) have been cited. These large differences in decay times can conceivably be explained by the use of different detectors with different rise times - since this will determine the detected top luminance and hence the decay time.

The degree of oscillation has also been characterized by uniformity figures (UF), i.e. the quotient between the darkest and the brightest phase of the cycle. Thus, a low UF corresponds to a 'high' degree of oscillation. These measurements, in contrast to those of decay times, are performed in an illuminated workroom, and the UFs measured are thus related to both the brightness control and the work room lighting. The UFs of single dots presumably correspond to the oscillation experienced by the fovea, (Läubli et al., 1981). Other indices are also used to quantify time variations, such as the flicker index (IBM, 1984). This is defined as F= A/B, where B is the time average of the luminance, and A is the time average of that fraction of the luminance that exceeds B.

Top luminance. The measurement of the top luminance (luminance during steady state, i.e. during excitation) requires instruments capable of recording luminances within 100 ns. Fellmann and coworkers (1982) examined eight VDTs. Two 'extreme' VDTs were described with mean luminances of 40 and 38 cd/m^2 respectively, and top luminances of about 75 and 700 cd/m^2 respectively. Decay times (100% to 10% of recorded luminance) were more than 20 ms and about 2 ms respectively. These recorded decay times are in excess of those reported by Clinton Corp.

Nylén & Bergqvist (1986) found that a P$_{31}$ phosphor (with a decay time of 11 us) had a calculated top luminance of about 65 000 cd/m^2, based on a mean luminance of 50 cd/m^2. For a slow phosphor ('amber'), the decay time was in excess of 16 ms, and the top luminance was about 200 cd/m^2. It should be emphasized that these calculated top luminances were based on the same total (energy) output.

The blitz phenomenon. Operators working with positive image screens, and also viewing customers or other objects above the screen (e.g. in bank offices or travel bureaux) sometimes perceive a brightly shining horizontal line when their gaze moves downwards on the screen. A tentative explanation of this phenomenon ('blitz') has been offered by Nylén (1985): The operator's (vertical) gaze velocity is similar to the vertical sweep velocity of the VDT. Thus, the operator's gaze may follow the 'front' of the illumination down the screen, and therefore a luminance considerably higher than the average screen luminance is seen.

This 'blitz' phenomenon was observed with a fast phosphor (P$_{31}$), but not with a slow ('amber'). This is in accordance with the fast phosphor's higher contrast between top and mean luminance (see Fig. 3).

Flicker. Variations in the luminance during one refresh period can be experienced as flicker. The critical flicker fusion (CFF) is defined as the frequency at which (with 100% modulation), no flicker is recognizable (Kalsbek & Umbach, 1982).

In a field survey (Turner, 1982), 12% of examined VDTs showed flicker. In another survey, no flicker was observed on any examined screen. However, 68%

of the operators complained about flicker (Stammerjohn, 1981). Flicker perception is dependent on a number of other parameters apart from the refresh rate, for example, polarity, screen luminance, room illumination, degree of oscillation, contrast as well as on whether foveal or perifoveal vision is utilized and on individual sensitivity (Grandjean, 1980; National Research Council, 1983; Rogowitz, 1984; Stammerjohn, 1981). The variations in luminance during one refresh period can be perceived as a flicker. In principle, increasing the luminance by a factor of 10 will increase the highest frequency at which flicker is noticeable with 10 Hz (Bauer & Cavonius, 1982; National Research Council, 1983). Bauer (1984) recorded the CFF values for 30 observers. With a luminance of 80 cd/m^2, the CFF varied between 55 and 88 Hz, with a mean of 73 Hz. With decreased VDT luminance and increased ambient illuminance, flicker was noticed at a larger angle (Isensee & Bennett, 1983). Experiments by Nishiyama and colleagues (1982) suggest that the CFF declines after exposure to 30 or 60 Hz.

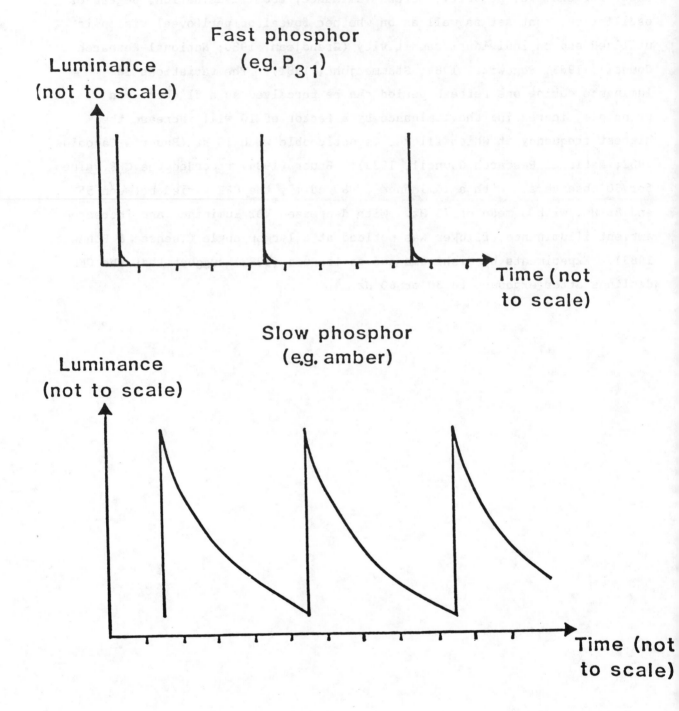

Fig. 3: The real time appearance of the luminance of a fast (above) and a slow (below) phosphor.

Low-frequency modulation (periods of several seconds) of the flicker may appear due to the oscillation caused by interference with the room lighting. A fixed synchronisation between the CRT refresh rate and the mains - especially with a 180° phase shift - may eliminate this phenomenon (Guekos & Ulmi, 1983).

Flicker may adversely affect the visual comfort of the operator - and thus possibly cause asthenopia symptoms. Effects on visual reading performance per se have not been established (National Research Council, 1983). Visible flicker may cause an adaptive overload of the eye, since the retina will be repetitively overexposed (Cakir et al., 1980; Iwasaki & Kurimoto, 1986) although this has been criticized (see National Research Council, 1983). A 'flicker discomfort rating' (Isensee & Bennett, 1983) increased with VDT luminance and was slightly reduced for moderate VDT luminances by increased ambient luminances. Iwasaki & Kurimoto (1986) measured small fluctuations in accommodation in an experiment using a flickering light (not a screen). They suggested that watching a flicker may affect this accommodation fluctuation, and that this possibly includes also non-percieved flicker.

Rogowitz (1984) has presented a method for measuring perceived flicker on VDTs, including determination of the perceived flicker frequency. The author suggests that a precise criteria for 'flicker-free VDT' be developed - for example, "flicker-free to 95% of the population up to 85% contrast".

Further work is currently being done on methods to measure perceived flicker, in terms of CFF. Suggested methods require data on screen luminance, refresh rate and screen size (Eriksson, 1986; Farrell & Moran, 1986, Zülch et al., 1986).

Jitter. Time variation in the position of display characters can sometimes be observed. This phenomenon is due to the improper variations in the magnetic fields used to deflect the electron beam.

These time variations may have a frequency of 0.03 - 0.5 Hz. In eight VDTs examined, considerable jitter was found in four (Fellmann et al., 1982). Subjective evaluations found three makes of VDTs with good stability, and the other five with 'continuous trembling'. Jitter is in principle harmless but may be irritating and tiring.

Afterglow. Some phosphors, notably those used for radar display, have a considerable afterglow, i.e. the character luminance decreases very slowly, and is perceived for several refresh periods after the corresponding pixels are no longer irradiated. With sufficiently fast phosphors, normally used for VDTs, this phenomenon should not be observable (IBM, 1984).

5.2.3.2 Structure of screen characters

Characters and symbols. The character image may be composed either of strokes or dots. Examples of both image systems occur frequently. The information processing techniques may be different in stroke as compared with dot characters (National Research Council, 1983). Dot matrix presentation has been claimed to be superior for legibility (Fellmann et al., 1982). The fonts used in VDT representations are quite different from many established fonts in printed text, thus there may be a conflict between acceptability (expected notions of character appearances), identifiability and distinctness. Optimal font design is of particular importance for noncontextual presentations (Bouma, 1982).

Resolution and character matrix. A visible raster scan (series of horizontal lines) or line pattern decreases legibility. This will dictate a minimum of scanning line density, e.g. 729 or 1029 (obviously depending also on screen size) (National Research Council, 1983).

Matrix sizes vary from 5 x 7, 7 x 9, etc. Increasing the matrix from 5 x 7 to 7 x 9 will increase reading performance (14% improvement in reaction time, 10% decrease in errors in one study) (Haubner & Kokoschka, 1983). A 7 x 9 dot matrix is necessary for presentation of both upper-case and lower-case letters (Campbell & Durdent, 1983).

The optimum size of the characters is dictated both by sufficient size for identification and by not being too large, since otherwise too few characters could be read simultaneously in the fovea (see, for example, Bouma, 1982). The character height has an optimum for reading performance of some 20-28 minutes of arc which means about 3.8 mm at 60 cm distance. Some recommendations give somewhat different optimal height for different work tasks (text, single characters).

Resolution (related to the width of a single spot) and addressability (related to spot separation) are in principle independent parameters of a CRT screen. Matching these to each other and to human contrast sensitivity is related to improved performance (Murch & Beaton, 1986).

Spacing and legibility of words. Acceptable symbol line spacing is determined by the eye saccade movements. The distance between symbol lines should increase with an increasing line length, with a minimum of a 2° return trajectory of the line saccade (line angle). To meet this, vertical orientation of a full page screen (e.g. with a 4:3 aspect) or a two-column presentation in horizontal orientation can be used (Bouma, 1982).

Sharpness and blur. In principle, the luminance is not constant across a single dot, but has a variable luminance distribution across any scan path of the dot. Techniques for evaluating sharpness include edge response and modulation transfer function.

The Modulation Transfer Function (MTF) is the Fourier transform of this line spread function. The MTF is a useful concept in analysing contrast, resolution, jitter, etc. (Banbury, 1982; National Research Council, 1983; Murch & Beaton, 1986).

Using an edge response technique, the sharpness of the characters can be characterized by the slope of the luminance across the character contour. This slope has been measured for five VDTs of different makes with negative polarity (Fellmann et al., 1982): at maximum luminance, the slopes varied between 63 and 350 cd/m^2, per mm and between 37 and 127 cd/m^2, per mm at the 'preferred' luminance. A VDT with good characteristics had a luminance slope of 116 cd/m^2, per mm, while a bad VDT had a slope of 37 cd/m^2, per mm (at preferred luminances). Sharpness was poor according to subjective evaluations (10 subject) for two of the eight VDT makes (Fellmann et al., 1982).

5.2.3.3 Luminance of screen information and workroom lighting

Polarity and general luminance. Negative polarity means light or irradiated characters on a dark, non-irradiated background. The opposite is positive polarity. A positive polarity screen will have an average luminance of 2-2.5 times that of a negative polarity screen (National Research Council, 1983). If the adaptation of the eye is determined by the average luminance, a positive polarity screen will imply a somewhat higher (about 15%) visual acuity. However, this has been criticized, on the suggestion that the adaptation is not based on the average, but on the higher luminance (IBM, 1984; National Research Council, 1983).

It has been suggested that transient adaptation glare may cause transient changes in pupil size when alternately viewing positive and negative polarity areas, as when looking alternatively at a document and the screen. This was based on experimental results using a slide projector (Cakir et al., 1980). However, the study was criticized on the ground that the response may have been due to the brief dark periods between the slides (National Research Council, 1983). Furthermore, adaptation is presumably sufficiently fast on the neural level for the operator not to notice the change (Campbell & Durdent, 1983). An immediate change-over between opposite polarities did result in a prolonged reaction time, compared to using the same polarity. However according to Taylor & McVey (1984), with a delay of 0.5 seconds, this prolonged reaction time did not materialize.

There may be other potential benefits of a higher luminance (increase in visual depth, increase in visual acuity, less contrast with surroundings, etc.). This is supported by the findings of Knave and colleagues (1985b), where large luminance ratios between the screen and the manuscript were associated with more asthenopia. Positive polarity may reduce the appearance of discomfort glare and diffuse reflections (Campbell & Durdent, 1983; Radl, 1982), which then reduces the measures necessary in workstation design, and requires less stringent workroom lighting restrictions [see comments by the National Board of Occupational Safety and Health, Sweden (1985b)]. According to Bauer (1986a, b), a positive polarity screen will perform better in a well-lit office, since it is less vulnerable to diffuse or specular reflexions. Zwahlen & Kothari (1986) suggested that either polarity is acceptable, provided that a sufficient character-background luminance contrast is provided.

In an experimental set up, positive polarity gave a higher test performance (letter transcribing) and a higher visual comfort rating, and was preferred by 19 of the 24 subjects (two having no preference and three preferred negative polarity) (Radl, 1982). Similar findings were made by Bauer & Cavonius (1982), where error rates were lower with positive polarity. In this experiment, 22 of the 23 subjects preferred positive polarity (one preferred negative polarity). The dependence on polarity may also be related to tasks, as suggested by Külne and colleagues (1986).

The flicker threshold will, however, be increased with increasing average luminance. A refresh rate of 50 Hz is not acceptable for positive polarity and a refresh rate of 100 Hz for positive polarity has been recommended by Bauer & Cavonius (1982). This does appear somewhat excessive; data from Bauer (1984) and practical experience suggest that a compromise (with phosphor type etc.) may be in the vicinity of 80-85 Hz.

Character stroke width should be somewhat wider for positive polarity according to the European Computer Manufacturers Association (1984).

A literature review on the issue of polarity (Herring & Berns, 1984) shows a preference for positive polarity compared to negative, by the majority of workers questioned. A similar conclusion was made by the Institut de Recherche en Santé et en Sécurité du Travail du Québec (1984), who concluded that "In view of these considerations, the group favors the use of positive-contrast screens provided that the flicker problem is solved." A different view is however taken by others: "Opinion is divided on the subject of image polarity, that is whether there are significant visual advantages in displays of positive polarity (dark symbols on light background) over displays of negative polarity (light symbols on a dark background). However, when these polarities are tested, there is little human factor advantage of one polarity over the other for most applications and operators." (IBM, 1984)

The diversity of opinion on polarity may in part be related to different implicit assumptions. Some experiments have been performed in experimental conditions of optimal light conditions (for each presentation). Others argue that realistic tests should not be made under optimal conditions, but under realistic conditions with, for example, reflexions from office lighting. It has been suggested (e.g. by Bauer, 1986b) that under such real conditions, the advantages of positive polarity are manifested. A second problem is to

discriminate the issue of polarity per se (i.e. whether the text is brighter
than the background or reverse) from that of the average screen brightness.
Reviewed literature is not always clear on this point. Most arguments for a
positive polarity screen appear to dwell mainly on screen brightness.
Finally, this debate is centred on monochromatic screens. Involved factors
are different and largely unknown when multicolour screens are concerned (see
further below).

Workroom illumination. Proper illumination is necessary for reading both
the screen and source documents. Recommendations for workroom illumination,
however, show considerable variations. For general office environments,
recommendations vary between 75 and 1600 lux. For VDT workplaces,
recommendations are considerably lower, often in the range of 100-500 lux
(Stammerjohn, 1981). Thus, there is an apparent conflict between illumination
on the source documents and on the screen, often solved by a low workroom
light level and additional lighting at the source document.

Subjects allowed to adjust the workroom illumination normally selected
illuminances of 200-600 lux. Turner (1982) found that workroom illumination
was less than 250 lux for 31%, 250-500 lux for 63% and more than 500 lux for
6% of the workplaces. A median of about 400 lux was reported by Von Kiparski
(1984). Higher levels were found by Stammerjohn (1981) with a median of
500-700 lux. Furthermore, the majority (53% and 63%) were satisfied with
workstation and background illumination. Knave and coworkers (1985b) observed
that workroom illumination was about 300 lux for VDT-operators, and 500 lux
for controls. (All VDT-operators used negative polarity screens.)

In data entry work, source illumination was 550 lux, compared to 430 lux
for conversational work, and 500-800 lux for non-VDT workers (Läubli et al.,
1981).

Contrasts between screen and the surroundings. There are several
definitions of contrast; a ratio $C_r = L_o/L_b$, or $C = (L_o-L_b)/L_b$, or
the modulation $(L_o-L_b)/(L_o+L_b)$, where L_o is the object luminance and
L_b is the background luminance. Data below, however, are presented as they
appear in the literature, thus often as the ratio C_r.

Contrasts have been suggested to be limited to 1:3 between the screen and the surroundings for the near field and 1:10 for the far field (Dainoff, 1982b). However, less restricted limits (up to 1:20) showed similar reading performances in one study (Haubner & Kokoschka, 1983). A ratio of 1:20 was associated with increased asthenopia by Knave and coworkers (1985b), especially for screen-manuscript differences. Sauter and colleagues (1983b), however, found no relationship between comfort and contrasts.

Turner (1982) found that 33% of work sites exceeded the near-field recommendation 1:3 (screen-source). For screen-background, near-field, 54% exceeded this recommendation. The far-field recommendation of 1:10 was exceeded in 24% of cases. Near-field contrasts noted by Fellmann and coworkers (1982) varied between 1:1 and 1:28 (negative polarity). Screen-source contrasts varied between 1:8 and 1:25, while screen-frame contrasts were between 1:1 and 1:8. Unsuitable colours on VDT boxes were frequently found, and could affect visual performance. Very high contrasts were noted by Läubli and coworkers (1981): 1:21-26 (near-field) and about 1:300 (far field). Von Kiparski (1984) found that 30% of a large investigated group had a manuscript-screen ratio of 20:1 or higher.

Reflections and discomfort glare. Reflections can be either specular (mirror-like) or diffuse. Here, only specular reflections are considered.

The virtual image, which may appear, will be located behind the screen. For example, reflection of the operators face will typically lie about 22 cm behind the screen. Different accommodation levels are in principle required for the screen text and the image; this may be annoying and cause possibly discomfort (National Research Council, 1983).

Glare can be defined as discomfort glare or disability glare, the latter being discussed below. It causes discomfort without immediate effects on reading performance. It may be direct from bright luminance objects or reflected from keyboard key, etc., (Stammerjohn et al., 1981).

In one field survey by Stammerjohn and coworkers (1981), 46 of 53 workstations investigated had potential discomfort glare due to luminance levels of up to 2 100 cd/m^2 from windows or lighting. In the same study, 80%

of the VDT-operators compared with 62% of the controls reported glare
problems. Isensee & Bennett (1983) found there was a decreased discomfort
glare rating with increased screen luminance, and lower ambient illuminance.

Brightness of irradiated screen areas. For negative polarity, adjusted
character luminances vary between 7 and 160 cd/m^2 (Bräuninger et al., 1982;
Grandjean, 1980; Gunnarsson & Söderberg, 1983). Preferred adjusted character
luminances in one field study were 31 cd/m^2 (range 23 - 42 cd/m^2 - with
the lower values obtained for a VDT with a fast phosphor) (Bräuninger et al.,
1982). Another study by Takahashi and colleagues (1984), indicated a preferred
character brightness of about 27 cd/m^2, decreasing to some 22 cd/m^2 at the
end of the 2-2.5 h session. In one field study, 70% of VDT-operators
complained about character brightness (Stammerjohn et al., 1981).

Screen constrasts and disability glare. Reflected diffuse glare determines
the luminance of the nonirradiated screen areas (background in negative
polarity, characters in positive polarity). Nonirradiated area luminances of
some 1-50 cd/m^2 have been reported. For the higher range, this may cause a
reduced contrast and disability glare, which directly interfers with reading
performance (Fellmann et al., 1982; Grandjean, 1980; Haubner & Kokoschka, 1983;
Stammerjohn et al., 1981).

Character-background contrasts among data entry workers were 2:1, and 9:1
among conversational mode workers. The latter type of work apparently led to
the operator adjusting the controls to predominantly screen viewing (Läubli et
al., 1981). Other field studies show varying contrasts (range 2:1 - 30:1)
(Grandjean, 1980; Haubner & Kokoschka, 1983; Smith, M.J., 1982).

A VDT with good characteristics had a screen contrast of 0.13
($C_r = L_o/L_b$), while a bad VDT had a contrast of 0.43 (preferred
luminance settings) (Fellmann et al., 1982). The preferred contrast also
increases with decreasing background luminance as well as with decreasing room
illumination (Haubner & Kokoschka, 1983).

The contrast between the background luminance near to a character and that
of the character was determined (for the letter U) for some VDTs. The near
background luminances were between 17% and 82% of the character luminance for

maximum luminance and between 13% and 45% for preferred luminances (Fellmann et al., 1982).

Kokoschka (1986) recently presented data indicating that "inner contrasts", i.e. contrasts between character pixels and non-character pixels within the characters (e.g. inside the letter 'o'), are more crucial than "outer contrasts".

The visual reading field is dependent on the contrast. Low contrasts have no effect on foveal word recognition, but have an impact on the parafoveal word recognition. For a contrast of 0.90, about 80% of the words were correctly recognized, compared to less than 50% correct words at a contrast of 0.12. (Positive polarity, contrast defined as $C_+ = (L_B-L_C)/L_B$; L_B = background, L_C = character luminance) (Bouma, 1982). The visual field extension may be of importance for contextual reading. Similar results have also been reported by (Timmers et al., 1982), where both errors and response times were increased with decreasing contrast. These studies were performed with paper documents.

Campbell & Durdent (1983) presented arguments for a broad range of contrasts, adjustable for individual preference. The main argument was that "almost full visual acuity can be achieved over a wide range of contrast".

In one field study by Stammerjohn and coworkers (1981), 62% of VDT-operators complained about screen brightness. Reflected glare was present in 17% of all workstations at a level sufficient to make reading difficult, since the contrasts between bright and dark areas were considerably reduced.

Screen colour. There are few definite data to support the choice of a specific phosphor/screen colour (Grandjean et al., 1984; National Research Council, 1983; Rosenbaum, 1981; Sivak & Woo, 1983) and, despite some general and rather vague suggestion of green-yellow as the best, this issue is often considered secondary to other display parameters (National Research Council, 1983; Rosenbaum, 1981; Shahnavaz, 1982). Recently, Wichansky (1986) suggested that although white, green or orange gives the same legibility (negative polarity), green could cause annoying after-images. White is preferred for

presentations using mixed polarities and for positive polarity screens. At
far viewing distances, green or orange are seen at further distances, while
white results in fewer legibility errors. The possible impact of phosphor
colour on screen contrasts should be considered (Timmers et al., 1982).
Colour filters are not to be recommended according to Radl (1982).

Most phosphors hitherto used for display purposes have a yellowish green
colour, both during steady state (excitation) and during decay. Some common
phosphors have a white colour (e.g. P_4, P_{40}), and orange or amber colours
do also occur (National Research Council, 1983; Paulsson et al., 1984). From
the standpoint of colour blindness and colour stereopsis, saturated red and
blue colours are not to be recommended (Van Nes, 1986; Verriest et al., 1986).

The use of multiple colours for ease of scanning is increasing, but the
designs have not always been optimal. Different colours should be used to
increase proper emphasis. For example, red has a stronger emphasis than
green, and should thus be used only for work important for the scanning
process. The use of colours for information purposes is seldom optimal, since
the colour discrimination ability of human beings is rather limited (Engel,
1982; Radl, 1982; Smith, 1986; Van Nes, 1986).

Multicolour (shadow-mask) VDT presentations may pose problems for people
with colour-defective vision. To a lesser degree, older people and people
with only basic education may experience greater difficulties as well
(Verriest et al., 1986). In a study on screen mask design, delimit blocks by
colour alone did not improve performance, while spacing did. Spacing and
colour delimination was however far superior to any one method alone according
to Haubner & Benz (1984).

5.2.4   Work environment

A number of environmental characteristics are relevant to a discussion of
possible health effects of working on a VDT. They will be defined and briefly
discussed in this section, mainly as to common parameter values. Their
possible health effects are discussed in section 5.3 covering health
implications of VDT work.

General physical characteristics of the office environment include such parameters as temperature, humidity and floor resistance. Physicochemical characteristics include measurements or air ions, air contaminants and some other relevant parameters. Illumination characteristics are related to several display characteristics and are described in pp. 48-62.

Workstation design is of primary importance for musculoskeletal comfort. A number of texts exist on suggestions and recommendation for good workstation design, both in general and as applied to VDT workstation. In this section, a discussion relevant to VDT workstation designs will be given - primarily on operators position at the workstation.

5.2.4.1 <u>General physical characteristics</u>

<u>Room temperature and humidity</u>. In an epidemiological study by Knave and coworkers (1985b), the room temperatures experienced by VDT-operators and controls were 24.1^{o}C and 24.8^{o}C respectively. In another study by Cato Olsen (1981), the temperature of some VDT offices was about 22°C.

In the study by Knave and coworkers (1985b), the mean relative humidity for some 400 VDT-operators was 36.5% (34.8% for approximately 150 controls). In a Bergen study, the relative humidity was 'consistently' below 30% (with outdoor weather cold and dry) (Cato Olsen, 1981). In another study, two-thirds of the operators complained about dry air (at 30-40% humidity), (Smith, M.J., 1982). Very low relative humidity is generally found in northern areas in wintertime, when the difference between the warm indoor and the cold outdoor temperature is large.

In principle, there is a relationship between relative humidity and body potentials, since body charges are eliminated much faster in humid than in dry conditions. There is also an inverse relationship between the electrostatic field from the VDT and relative humidity.

<u>Floor covering and resistance</u>. In one study by Knave and coworkers (1985b), women tended to use rooms furnished with fitted carpets to a greater degree than men (86% versus 61%). The floor resistance was generally very high, 9 700 Mohm for men, and 8200 Mohm for women. In neither parameter was

there any difference between VDT operators and controls doing similar types of work.

5.2.4.2 Physicochemical characteristics

Measurements of ion concentrations in air. In a study of about 400 VDT workstations and 150 controls (Nylén et al., 1984), 'light' ions in air were measured both close to the operator's face and in the workroom at least a few metres from the VDT and the operator (or the control). Both positive and negative ion levels were generally significantly increased at both positions, compared to the controls. 'Exposed' levels varied between 0.95×10^8 and 2.62×10^8 ions/m^3, while 'control' values were between 0.68×10^8 and 1.05×10^8 ions/m^3. There was a difference between levels for men and for women – all men 0.55–1.73×10^8, and all women 1.00–2.40×10^8 ions/m^3. Charry (1986) found a small decrease in air ions (both positive and negative) close to VDTs with electrostatic fields. It should be noted that the variations found both by Nylén and coworkers (1984) and Charry (1986) are small compared to variations due to other factors (e.g. ventilation) and within normal ranges found in offices.

Air particulates. The particles of interest in this discussion are primarily the 'accumulation mode particles'; i.e. particles between less than 0.1 and 1 um diameter. These particles are normally found to be due to the coagulation of smaller, primary particles.

Cato Olsen (1981) examined the total mass of suspended particles in the air of some VDT offices sampling only particles less than 10 μm size (aerodynamic diameter). The range of 60 measurements was 10 – 450 μg/m^3. All values above 150 μg/m^3 were found following periods of cigarette smoking. Non-smoking areas had a range of 12 – 40 μg/m^3. These measurements show general agreement with data found in University Park Press (1979). Charry (1986) did not find any influence of electrostatic fields from VDTs on concentrations of respirable air particulates in the room, nor on removal of cigarette smoke.

These particles normally carry charges due to the presence of charging mechanisms. One such important mechanism is interaction between these particles and air ions.

Air contaminants. The sources of the aerosol constituents are diverse.
Generally compounds such as sulfur dioxide reaction products, hydrocarbon
oxidation products, nitrates, etc. will be found present in many areas, but
with the possibility of considerable geographical variations due to the
proximity of saline water, frequency of inversion phenomena, etc. Other
constituents depend on specific anthropogenic sources in the area (metals,
metal oxides, many organic compounds, etc.). (See a general review in
University of Park Press, 1979.) Furthermore, indoor sources may contribute
significantly to the indoor aerosol. One such major constituent is cigarette
smoke (see above).

In a study by Murray and coworkers (1981a), some chemical contaminants
were sampled at 136 workstations in three different sites. The levels of
carbon dioxide, carbon monoxide, formaldehyde and acetic acid were very low.
The major source of carbon monoxide was smoking.

The levels of polychlorinated biphenyls (PCB) have been measured in a few
VDT workplaces. Levels of 56-81 ng/m^3 were found, whereas only 0.5-1
ng/m^3 were found outside the building. Digernes and Astrup (1982) suggested
that the capacitor and transformer components of these VDTs may contain PCB,
and that the PCB levels found in these workplaces may have originated from
such VDT components. They did not, however, measure the PCB levels in
VDT-free rooms in the building. Another study did not reveal any differences
in PCB concentrations between VDT-offices, offices without VDTs and outdoor
levels (Nylén, 1984).

Benoit and coworkers (1984) discussed other possible indoor PCB sources
(fluorescent lamp ballast and caulking material) and suggested that PCB
emitted from VDTs was the result of previous deposits of ambient PCB on the
VDT, and subsequent evaporation when the VDT was operated, and thus heating
certain parts.

Aerosol deposition. In the absence of any electrostatic field, and in the
fairly calm office air, diffusion is probably the dominant transport mode of
these particles (size less than 1 μm). However, in the presence of an
electrostatic field, the electric mobility may influence the transport.
Particles 0.03 μm in size have a mobility of about 10^{-3} cm/s per V/cm (1 μm

particles have a mobility of some 10^{-5} cm/s per V/cm. Thus, particles in a field of about 10 kV/m would move at about 0.01 mm/s (1 µm size) to 1 mm/s (0.03 µm size) (Cato Olsen, 1981). These transport velocities do however appear small in comparison to ambient air velocities as measured at 100-140 mm/s by Knave and coworkers (1985b). The deposition of these particles on a surface (e.g. the face) is probably maintained until they are physically removed by washing, etc. (Cato Olsen, 1981).

The deposition of air particulates in two VDT offices has been measured by Cato Olsen (1981). A substrate was charged with a positive or negative potential, and placed at a distance from a VDT (with a positive potential). The impacted particles were counted in an electron microscope. The deposition appears to be related to the applied potentials, although the influence of either is less clear. The data do suggest the necessity of a charge on the substrate (thus on the operator) for excess deposition to occur, but this must be confirmed by further studies.

The insignificance of the transport velocity compared to ambient air velocities, the probable importance of substrate potential as well as some theoretical considerations, suggest that the potential charge of the substrate does mainly perform a 'trap' function rather than a 'transport' function, (see Ungethüm, 1984).

The particles deposited in the study referred to above (Cato Olsen, 1981) were examined as to size distribution and also subjected to limited chemical analysis. The total surface of the particles shows a maximum around 0.3 to 0.6 µm. Based on these data, it was estimated that a proportion of the aerosol submicron mass in a cubic metre of air will be deposited every hour on the face of the operator under the conditions prevailing at those offices (Cato Olsen, 1981). The chemical analysis of individual larger particles disclosed a relative abundance of the aluminium, silicon and calcium, followed by sodium, sulfur, chlorine, potassium and iron, and finally magnesium. The majority of these particles were however probably carbonaceous. In the smaller particles, an enrichment of sulfur and chlorine was found.

Radon deposition. In a recent experimental study, the Swedish National Institute of Radiation Protection (Bengtsson, 1986) has investigated the effect of high electrostatic fields at VDT workstations on the deposition of radon daughters on the face of the operator. On a yearly basis, and for a radon air concentration of 100 Bq/m^3, the radiation dose would increase by some 50-60%. The Institute concluded that this increase by itself was not so great as to be able to cause any skin changes.

5.2.4.3 General factors for workstation design

Dimensions of the operators. Some investigators have used existing standard body dimensions to estimate viewing distance and viewing angle from data on workstation configuration, see Murray and coworkers (1981b). This may lead to some error, however. In an experimental set up with adjustable display (height, distance and tilt) and keyboard (height and distance), the subjects had full freedom within the mechanical limits to adjust the workstation configuration for maximum comfort. The position of the eyes of these operators were compared to eye position of 'statistical subjects', using anthropometrical data based on the subjects height but with a standard posture. The real subjects tended to have their eyes about 10 cm closer than the 'statistical' subjects (Brown & Schaum, 1982).

Viewing distance. Viewing distances have been measured from the operators eyes to the screen, the keyboards and the manuscripts. The viewing angle, defined as angle below the horizontal line, to the screen has also been investigated. These data are of primary interest for vision correction (presbyopes) and for posture.

The viewing distances are in general further from the screen than from the source documents and keyboards. Mean values in the literature vary between 43 and 88 cm for eye to screen distances and between 47 and 53 cm for eye to document distances (Grandjean, 1980; Hünting et al., 1981; Knave et al., 1985b; Laville, 1982; Murray et al., 1981b; Shahnavaz, 1982). Eye to keyboard distances were closer than eye to manuscript distances. The latter were about 5 cm longer for VDT-operators than for controls, according to Knave and coworkers (1985b). These viewing distances vary considerably depending on the type of work, the adjustability of workstation configuration, individual variations, etc. Jaschinski-Kruza (1986) examined individuals with a far dark focus, and found that they preferred longer viewing distances than other individuals.

Viewing angles were examined by Murray and colleagues (1981b) (computed from a field study) and found to vary between nil and 30° or more. Men usually viewed at 21° - 30° while women tended to view at somewhat smaller angles, but generally within the 10° - 30° range. In an experimental set-up, the mean viewing angle, as adjusted by the subjects was 17° (Brown & Schaum, 1982). In another study by Grandjean and coworkers (1984), the preferred angle was between 4° and 14°. Optimal line of sight to the screen may be lower than previously thought. In one experiment (Kroemer & Hill, 1986), the preferred viewing angle was about 34° below horizontal. The authors suggest that if these data were confirmed, then workstation design should be rearranged to meet this viewing angle.

Work posture. Work posture investigations are of importance to determine adequacy of workstation design, in terms of the possibility of developing muscular discomfort.

Major factors for determining posture appear to be the job task and individual factors (dimensions) (Arndt, 1983; Miller & Suther, 1983), as well as attitudes, health (vision), habits and motivation (Arndt, 1983). There is an interaction between work posture and immobility and visual ergonomic factors such as glare - the latter may cause considerable restriction of posture flexibility.

In general, considerable variations were found in the postures of operators with different worktypes (Smith, A.B. et al., 1982). Conversational terminal workers had more lateral head rotation than data entry workers (Hünting et al., 1981). Traditional typists had more extreme postures as to their arms and hands in several respects than had habitual VDT workers.

There is a tendency for operators to sit in a reclined position with a tilted backrest (Läubli, 1986). This is to some degree in accordance with the reduction of muscular activity when reclining the thoracolumbar spine (Schüldt et al., 1986), but may have disadvantages, in restricting head and neck movability, which may be important in certain tasks. Thus, adjustability of workstations to encompass both reclining and upright position is justified (Läubli, 1986).

Furthermore, a comparison was made by Laville (1982) between 'simple data entry' and 'data ciphering and entry'. The former group had a larger homogeneity of posture than the latter. The average number of observed posture variants, during the observation period, was 2.6 compared with 13.6. Immobilization was not total in any group, but clearly higher in the simple data collecting group. This was presumably due to the operators glancing largely at a single element (document) and spending less time looking elsewhere or to the higher speed of the work, compared to that of the data ciphering operators.

Importance of flexibility. The results cited above should not be used to define a correct posture workstation design, for several reasons. First, differences as to the correct posture exist in the literature; secondly, individual dimensions vary considerably from the norm – especially when considering males and females or ethnic differences; thirdly, individual preferences may show considerable variations, as does work demand; and fourthly, fixing an optimal posture may lead to immobility.

An adjustable workstation appears to be of major importance. One example has been given by Sauter (1984), where the absence of a detachable keyboard was found to be associated with the increased occurrence of muscular pain. Murray and colleagues (1981b), suggested flexibility for seat height, backrest height and tension, keyboard height, screen height and angle. Workstations adjustable for individual settings should decrease muscular discomfort, compared to fixed settings (Grandjean et al., 1984). In the latter case, it was noted that "some of the preferred settings strongly differ from those recommended in many brochures and standards".

The need to move is based on several physiological events such as dynamic muscle contraction required for venous return, dynamic or static effort involved to avoid pain from muscle fatigue, skin discomfort at the point of contact with the chair, etc. An easily adjustable workstation leading to fewer discomforts, was also used easily and frequently for adjustments (Shute & Starr, 1984). The authors suggested that a high frequency of adjustments (flexibility) might be as important as providing a preferred setting.

5.2.5 <u>Contextual factors</u>

Certain operator characteristics will influence the incidence of reported health effects of VDT-operators. The differences between male and female reporting are apparent in some investigations, but other characteristics may also be of importance. Operator characteristics relating primarily to station design, such as body dimensions, are briefly discussed above (see p. 67).

The job design and the psychosocial environment have major influences on many of the reported health effects afflicting workers on VDTs. It is apparent that VDT operator-groups under study must also be characterized as to the type of work performed as well as the organization and social context of their work.

A description of interactions between the different aspects of psychosocial factors have been offered by the joint ILO/WHO report (1984). A summarizing figure from this report is given in Figure 4.

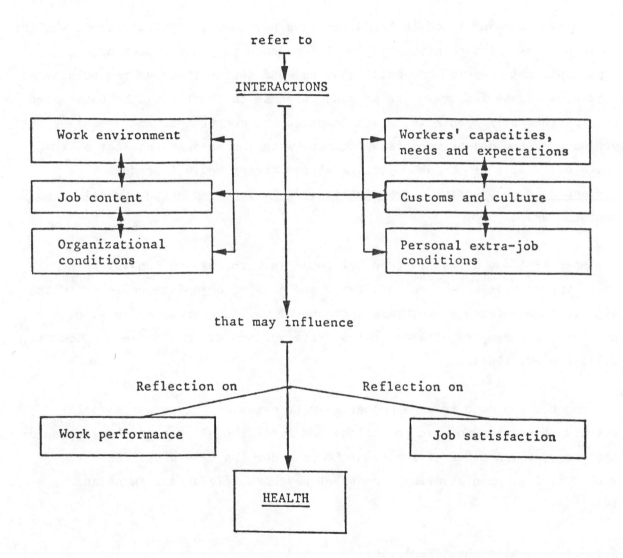

Fig. 4: Psychosocial factors at work. From ILO/WHO (1984).

This section will mainly concentrate on operator characteristics, which includes some aspects of workers' capacities, on job content and on some organizational conditions. Interactions with work environment and with some other factors will be discussed where appropriate. Influences as to job satisfaction will be mentioned where data are available. Influences on health care are discussed in section 5.3.

There are several models for discussing psychosocial influences of working on VDTs. One approach uses work conditions such as job requirement, organizational aspects and social aspects, and define these as the origins of objective stress factors. The persons response to these would be determined by a person-environment-fit, which compares the constraints and demands produced by the objective stress factors, with the need and ability of the operator. Misfit as to one objective stress factor would introduce a corresponding subjective stress factor (see National Research Council, 1983; Sauter, 1984).

Most of these stress factors are found in both VDT and non-VDT work. Their appearances depend on work types and design, organization, etc. With similar stress factors, VDT work and non-VDT work are expected to give generally the same results as to job satisfaction (National Research Council, 1983; Sauter, 1984).

Another approach is more concerned with dynamics - i.e. psychosocial effects of changes in work conditions. Many of the effects of changes may be temporary, which makes it important to consider the time aspect of VDT work-duration, when studying effects of psychosocial factors (Westlander, 1984).

5.2.5.1 Operator characteristics

Sex of the operator. In general, nonprofessional VDT-workers are predominantly women. In Canada, women constitute some 40% of the total work force, but up to 60-70% of the workers in jobs liable to be affected by the introduction of VDTs, such as clerical workers, typists, secretaries, telephone operators, tellers and reservation clerks (Labour Canada, 1982). In a Swedish study (Knave et al., 1985a), comprising 395 VDT-operators and 141 controls in office-type work, women amounted to 73 % of the subject group, which was not selected according to sex, but only as to all full-time employees at certain offices (newspaper, insurance, airline and post office). The predominance of women in many VDT workplaces is not necessarily true, however, of newspaper offices (see Knave et al., 1985a; Smith, A.B. et al., 1982).

The importance of this sex difference is reflected in the fairly consistent findings of higher discomforts and adverse health among women compared to men in comparable jobs (see further specific details for the various health effects in Knave et al. [1985a] and Evans [1986] for general comments).

The type of work may often, however, be quite different. In the Baltimore Sun study, females were more often found in data entry and clerical VDT-work (Smith, A.B. et al., 1982). In another field study (Hünting et al., 1981), 94% of data-entry workers were female, with only 50% of females in "conversational-type" work, involvinng both data-entry and data-acquisition operations. In a study in Japan, Kajiwara (1984) reported that women worked mainly with data entry and word processing, whereas men were more evenly distributed, and with a large proportion doing programming work. It is likely that one of the factors determining this difference in reported discomfort between men and women is the real differences in job tasks - possibly also within the coarse job designation of 'data entry', 'word processing', etc.

Age of the operator. The age of the operator appears to have an influence on several investigated health parameters. Sauter et al. (1983b) reported that age was negatively correlated with illness symptoms, but not correlated with mood disturbances. Similar effects of age on physical discomforts have been indicated by Ghingirelli (1982) and Starr (1984). Another study by Knave and coworkers (1985a) did not find any relationship between use and discomfort. However, age effects may differ depending on what illness symptom is considered, and its specific etiology. This may be pertinent to certain eye discomfort symptoms (see further pp. 88/89 and 113).

With increasing age and seniority, job tasks may differ, older people having more varied jobs with more control (McPhee, 1986). Age may also be

complicated by other work, such as household work and growing children, as
suggested by Ong & Phoon (1986). It is also possible, as indicated by McPhee
(1986) that reporting tendencies may differ between young and older people.

There are no general data on the age of VDT-operators. Specific data are,
when appropriate, referred to in the discussion of specific field studies. In
many studies the range of the age VDT-operators includes the full working age
(Knave et al., 1985a; Smith, A.B. et al., 1982). In contrast, the median age
was about 25 years (female) and about 30 years (male) for VDT-operators with
about 10% older than 40 years of age, in one study (Kajiwara, 1984).

Use of corrective eyewear. Some impairment of visual ability (glasses not
used or incorrect glasses used) may make VDT work more strenuous (see pp.
91-92). One such impairment is the presence of presbyopia, necessiting the
use of bi- or multifocal glasses. If such glasses are not adjusted for the
viewing distance involved (see below), the operator may have to choose between
suboptimal vision or an uncomfortable position. According to Böös and
coworkers (1985), an overcorrection of presbyopia was found among
VDT-operators (0.5 dioptres), taking into consideration the viewing distance.

Sauter and coworkers (1983b) found that VDT-operators with corrective
eyewear reported more eye and musculoskeletal discomfort than those without.
This was found in people wearing monofocal glasses and contact lenses, but not
in those using bifocal or trifocal glasses.

There are definite relationships between age and certain visual
characteristics, the most obvious one being presbyopia (see above). Another
well-known factor is light sensitivity [see further discussion by Meyer and
coworkers (1986)].

Personal characteristics. Personal habits may possibly influence symptoms
experienced during VDT work. Grandjean and coworkers (1984), suggested that
the use of medication, especially psychoactive drugs, might be a possible
confounder for certain eye symptoms. One suggested example is drugs that may
slow eye movements. In the investigation by Knave and colleagues (1985a),
users of several types of medicinal drugs (for anaemia, thyrotoxicosis,
nervous disorders and gastritis) reported more discomfort (eyes, muscles,

headache) and skin disorders than non-users. However, differences between VDT-exposed and controls were found to the same degree for non-drug users. Thus, the use of medicinal drugs does not explain such differences (Knave et al., 1985a).

Bolinder (1983) performed a field survey of hospital personnel (almost all female) using VDTs. Among the VDT-users (more than 8 h/week), smoking was more and physical exercise less common than among those who used VDTs occasionally (less than 8 h/week) or not at all. However, smoking or the use of alcohol did not correlate with subjective symptoms in the study by Knave and coworkers (1985a). Sauter and colleagues (1983b) analysed the possible relationships between personal characteristics and various discomforts and found very few significant relationships.

Education and other extra-job conditions. Few studies have explicitly given data on the education levels of VDT-workers. The education levels are presumably closely correlated with the type of job performed (the contrast, for example, between data entry and professional jobs), although large variations are to be expected between different types of workplaces.

In a study at a newspaper office in the USA by A.B. Smith and coworkers (1982) about 70% had at least a college level education. Furthermore, people with lower education were primarily found in 'eyes fixed mode' work (data entry or clerical). Knave and coworkers (1985a) found no correlation between education and subjective symptoms (the study investigated clerical workers only.)

Social aspects that might produce or affect strain are not limited to the workplace. Attention should be focused also on off-work situations, where possibly some differences in the situations of males and females are also of relevance. It is plausible that the women's responsibilities, extending into child care and the household, may produce more stress factors than in men.

Job dissatisfaction, mood disturbance and general illness were predicted from various social variables (the subjects almost exclusively females): married workers reported less strain, among both VDT and non-VDT users (Sauter, 1984). According to one recent study by Knutsson (1986), individuals with dyslexia (reading and writing difficulties) may experience increasing difficulties with the introduction of VDTs.

5.2.5.2 <u>Job content</u>

<u>Types of VDT-work</u>. The type of job performed is of major importance in
the occurrence of several symptoms, presumably due to some characteristics of
the work type which first, imposes certain physical restraints or patterns and
thus the possibility of muscular or visual strain, secondly, changes reporting
of subjective symptoms, and thirdly causes psychosocial stress factors.

In those field studies where job types of VDT and non-VDT workers have
been stated, terminology and definitions unfortunately vary. Several studies
differentiate between data entry and the "conversational" mode of operations,
or between data entry and data acquisition modes, and between clerical and
professional job categories. This type of classification thus centres on the
job content (see comments by Westlander, 1984), but does to some degree
contain an evaluation as to intensity and qualification demands. One widely
accepted classification of job types as noted below, was described by the
National Research Council (1983), and is based on the predominant mode of
operation:

1. <u>Data entry</u>: Information is keyed into the computer, often according to a
set format. Information may be noncontextual. Work pace is often high, with
few interruptions, little control of work speed and few opportunities for
decision making. The visual emphasis is on the source document.

2. <u>Data acquisition</u>: Data is read on the screen, thus with a high visual
emphasis on the screen. The input rate is medium, with some interruptions.
Work-speed control and decision-making opportunities vary. (telephone
operator is one such example.)

3. <u>Interactive communication</u> (conversational mode): This work mode involves
both data entry and data acquisition operations - thus conversational with the
VDTs. The input rate is medium and intermittent, with visual emphasis on
screen. Lags for processing occur, work-speed control and decision-making
opportunities vary. (Travel reservation clerks belong to this category.)

4. <u>Word processing</u>: This involves text entry, recall, searching, format
organization and corrections. The input rate is high but intermittent, with
visual emphasis shifting between the screen and the source document.

Interruptions are few, with some opportunities for speed control and decision making.

5. Programming, computer-assisted design and manufacturing: These jobs are often characterized as professional. The time spent at a VDT unit may vary. Input rate is low and intermittent, with visual emphasis on both the screen and documents. Interruptions are frequent, and there are major opportunities for work-speed control and decision making.

Other definitions and categorizations occur, but in many cases conform reasonably well with the definitions presented here (see Sauter, 1984; Wilkins, R., 1983). The job definitions in job types 1 to 4 (above) are commonly referred to as clerical in contrast to job type 5, which is classed as professional. Another field study by A.B. Smith and coworkers (1982) differentiated between 'eyes fixed mode' (data entry or clerical) and 'eyes shift mode' (conversational or professional) work types. 'Eyes fixed mode' was included in jobs with VDT being a major work component, in contrast to 'eyes shift mode' work.

It is possible that the definitions given above may be insufficient for precise work characterization. Laville (1982) found considerable differences as to both position and degree of immobilization between simple data entry and data ciphering and entry, although both could be classified as data-entry work (see the following subsection).

Such classification systems appear well suited for discussion on visual and postural factors, (see however the comments above). Different classifications of work may, however, be more relevant when discussing work psychology - primarily defined in terms of qualifications, intensity of work, etc. (Westlander, 1984).

5.2.5.3 Relationships between job content, work environment and display utilization. In one study by Läubli et al. (1981), the mean luminance on the source documents was considerably higher (163 cd/m^2) for data-entry work than for conversational work (108 cd/m^2), with reflexions being more prominent for data entry work. Apparently, the data-entry operators adjusted their lighting conditions primarily for the source documents, while the

conversational terminal operators aimed for good reading conditions on the
screen. In a field survey by Smith, A.B. and coworkers (1982), a positive
correlation was found between 'bothersome visual aspects of VDT as adjusted'
with'job attitude of demanding work'.

The time looking at the screen has been investigated in some studies.
Knave and coworkers (1985a) found no significant difference in total glance
time between data aquisition and interactive communication. The total glance
time was in this study between 0.9 and 1.6 h/day comprising between 14% and
22% of the total working time in the same day. Variations given are between
means of different workplaces. In 'simple data entry' (Laville, 1982), 70% of
the time was spent looking at the document, 18% at the screen, 10% at the
keyboard and 2% elsewhere. In 'data ciphering and entry', 30% of the time was
spent looking at the screen, 28% at the document, 15% at the keyboard and 27%
elsewhere. For computer-assisted design operators, in one study by Van der
Heiden and colleagues (1984), 50% of the working time was spent looking at the
screen.

Yamamoto & Noro (1986) investigated operators doing data-entry and data-
aquisition (search) tasks. Data-entry workers spent 28% of work looking at the
screen, 21% on the keyboard, 40% on documents and 10% elsewhere. There were
differences between experienced and inexperienced workers doing data-entry
work, in that the former spent a shorter time looking at a keyboard and a
longer time at the screen and elsewhere. There were no differences between
experienced and inexperienced operators doing search work, both spent more
than 99% of their time looking at the screen.

Screen glance may vary considerably, between 1 s (data entry), 6-8 s (word
processing) to 135 s (conversational) (Elias et al., 1982; Laville, 1982).
Glance frequencies also vary, from 12-18/min (data entry) to 8/min (word
processing) (Elias et al., 1982).

In one field study (Delvolé & Queinnec, 1983), document transcription was
studied. Glance sequences involving only screen and document remained fairly
steady (about 15/min) during the day, regardless of whether short or long
documents were processed. However, the frequency of glance sequences also
involving keyboards increased during that day, and was higher for long

documents. Thus, increased visual emphasis was given to keyboards during the day.

In an experimental set-up, the mean fixation time of experienced and inexperienced workers producing railway tickets was recorded. Fixation times differed between the two groups, but the results were not fully explainable by inexperienced workers needing longer fixation times (Graf et al., 1986).

VDT work per se may, however, introduce some specific stress factors, such as lag times, breakdown of equipment (Johansson & Aronsson, 1984) (see pp. 125-126), and dependency on software design. The last-mentioned can be described in terms like "learning the commands" (e.g. simplicity of commands, ease and control of changes), "presentation manner" (e.g. pagewise or roll-wise, control of 'turning pages'), "keeping track of position within information" (present 'state' of information) and "the user as an active participant" (e.g. keeping registers of certain information) (Waern & Rollenhagen, 1983; see also Kessel, 1984).

One study by Romano & Sonnino (1984) suggested that the use of a 'mask' arrangement of the data input functions for quick identification and access and fewer delayed responses resulted in increased efficiency and reduced stress of on-line input operations. Improvement could to some degree also be achieved without a mask, when an auditory signal suggesting readiness for new data input was used.

A summary list of 'desirable features of screen design' has been presented by Galitz (1984): 1) an orderly, clean, clutter-free appearance; 2) an obvious indication of what is being shown and what should be done with it; 3) expected information where it should be; 4) a clear indication of what is related to what; 5) plain simple language; 6) a simple way of finding what is in the system and how to get it out; 7) a clear indication of when an action could make a permanent change in the data or system operation. Based on these 'desirables' some general guidelines were presented, namely cohesive grouping of screen elements - in order to perceive identifiable pieces, e.g. by providing menu screens, and screens carrying only relevant information.

There has been considerable discussion and data on man/machine interaction and screen information design. A number of studies were presented at the conference on Work With Display Units in Stockholm, 12-15 May 1986. The reader is referred to the forthcoming published proceedings from this conference, as that topic is not fully covered in the present publication.[1]

5.2.5.4 <u>Organizational conditions</u>

<u>Duration of VDT work</u>. The time (h/week) spent by operators at a VDT workstation is obviously dependent on a number of factors, and it is impossible to generalize. A few samples only will be mentioned. In one field study of a newspaper office by Smith, A.B. and coworkers (1982), the mean working time was 21.7 h/week, with a range of 1-64 h/week. It should be noted that the time spent at a VDT workstation may not correspond to the time actually spent working with the VDT. In the investigation by Knave and colleagues (1985a), the time working with VDTs was about 60%, and the time looking at the VDTs was about 15% of the total working time (clerical workers, various offices, a few data-entry workers).

In the Canadian Labour Congress study (1982) field survey data were presented on the frequency of eye, muscle and stress problem composites with varying hours per day of VDT work. For all three (composites of) variables, the frequencies were fairly stable up to 4 h work/day. Increasing the daily work period to 5 h or more produced an increase in all three problem composites. Similar results were reported by Wallin and coworkers (1983). These results were apparently not evaluated as to type of work, which may have differed across the workers with different work durations, and which may thus be a strong confounding factor. This is suggested by the data of Knave and colleagues (1985a).

One observation made by Stellman and coworkers (1986) was that operators who worked full-time at VDTs (in contrast with those working only part-time) had their jobs organized in such a way that they seldom left the workstations and moved around. Full-time VDT workers were also those who reported more muscle and eye discomforts compared to part-time VDT workers (as well as compared to non-VDT workers). In the paper by Evans (1986), the responses to 'often eyestrain' and 'often painful/stiff neck or shoulder' were more frequent among those working a longer time at VDTs.

------

1 Publication is anticipated early in 1987.

Worry over health hazards (e.g. due to 'radiation') has increased during the last years among those working extensively at VDTs, but decreased for those working only a limited time on VDTs (Wright, 1986), a finding which was true also for certain discomforts such as musculoskeletal symptoms.

Duration of work tasks and rest periods. Breaks in the working period are necessary, and will contribute to comfort. These breaks may amount to doing alternative work, stretch breaks, coffee and lunch breaks as well as exercise breaks. The optimal pattern of breaks has not been fully documented, however. It is possible that short, informal breaks may do more to alleviate symptoms of muscle and eye troubles. This assumption is based on the study by Turner (1982). These findings were, however, criticized by Dainoff (1982a), on the grounds that a decreasing incidence of blurred vision may be more related to formal longer breaks. The suggestion of informal short breaks for alleviating muscle complaints is in accordance with the discussion of immobility as a causative factor for muscle pain. Wennberg & Voss (1986) made a laboratory investigation of videocoding (very intensive VDT work), and indicated that frequent breaks made work less strenuous, and resulted in a somewhat increased work speed and quality.

According to the paper by Delvolé & Queinnec (1983), lunch breaks did decrease the frequency of keyboard glances when doing short-time jobs, but not when involved in long-time jobs. In a Japanese study by Kajiwara (1984), consecutive operations were most often found in the 0.5 - 1 h or more than 3 h brackets (women worked more with the short-time jobs, men - with a higher proportion of programmers - more with the long-time jobs). In all 30-40% had a rest period after each work task, lasting normally for 10-25 min but, 20% were seldom able to take a rest after the work task.

Stress factors related to organizational aspects. In a report by the National Research Council (1983), some objective stress factors have been suggested, based on theoretical considerations and some circumstancial evidence only. They include workers' control, participation in job decisions, predictability and controllability of the work, work complexity, role ambiguity, threat of unemployment, quantitative workload, overload due to deadlines and occurred delays, worker's responsibility, role conflicts and social support. Comments on person-environment fit on these stress factors are found in the report. Many of these stress factors are found in other reports reviewed (Dainoff, 1982b; Sauter, 1984; Smith, M.J. et al., 1981; Smith, M.J. et al., 1982).

Organizational factors may be associated with VDT work as distress sources. Some specific organizational factors have been suggested: 1) lack of worker participation in VDT-implementation; 2) inadequate employee training; 3) job security issues (downgrading, advancement, job loss); 4) monitoring of employee performance and supervisory style; and 5) the presence of incentive pay schemes (Smith, M.J. et al., 1981). In a study of 222 VDT-workers, job autonomy was inversely related to VDT working-time. Data-entry workers also had less job autonomy than word processors. However, job autonomy did not correlate with discomfort (Pot et al., 1986).

In one study by Aronsson (1984), changes in qualification demands were noted in different hierarchial groups in an office. Demands concerning 'intensity' (concentration, vigilance, endurance, etc.) were increasing for low-echelon workers, whereas high-echelon workers did not note any changes. Demands concerning 'productivity' (responsibility, competence, etc.) and 'cooperation' (contact, dependency on others, etc.) did not change appreciably for any group. The author speculates whether the higher influence in high-echelon groups has determined the system appearances, or whether this is an effect of computerization of the high-echelon group's task being less complete. In general, higher intensity demands and routine work reduced user control and mental involvement (Aronsson, 1984; Johansson & Aronsson, 1984).

Social aspects. Several social aspects of VDT work have been studied, such as interaction between distance to neighbours and social contact or isolation. Some office worker data in the Canadian Labour Congress study (1982), reported that distances to coworkers were 'about right' for 59% and 'too crowded' for 34%. (Note that these data refer only to physical distance - and its possible influence on stress.) In another study, coworker satisfaction was significantly higher among VDT- than among non-VDT-workers (Travers & Stanton, 1984).

Job design-related stress factors. In one field study by Hünting and coworkers (1981) of two groups of bank clerks (one utilizing VDTs), differences were found as to variety; 'this work is varied' versus 'with this work one always has to do the same thing', with less variety found among VDT users. There were some differences on quantitative and qualitative overload (both less for VDT-operators), but no differences for task feedback or cooperation.

In another field study by Smith, A.B. and coworkers (1982), VDT users reported an intermittent work pace with more lulls than the controls had. Increasing the VDT work-duration (hours/week) was associated with decreased job autonomy, but also with a decreasing backlog of work and less work pressure. Increased VDT working-times have been related to higher levels of boredom, fatigue, monotony and work being specified in detail, but also to higher job satisfaction (Dainoff, 1982b).

'Eyes fixed mode' workers reported greater clarity in work definition, lesser job autonomy, lesser backlogged quantities of work and less work pressure. 'Eyes shift mode' workers reported a greater quantity of backlogged work and heavier work pressure (Smith, A.B. et al., 1982).

Clerical VDT workers have in some studies reported an increasing feeling of being dequalified by VDT work (compared to their old work), less meaningful jobs, greater fear of being replaced, faster work pace, and less control than professional VDT workers or non-VDT workers (Dainoff, 1982b; Smith, M.J. et al., 1982). In different workplaces, clerical VDT workers have indicated both more supervisory and less supervisory control, both less and more peer cohesion, both lower and higher work pace than the controls (Smith, M.J. et al., 1982).

There does not appear to be any fundamental differences between VDT and non-VDT jobs per se in certain psychosocial parameters. Examples of similarities between VDT and non-VDT work as to 'attitude', 'interest' and 'satisfaction' are found (Knave et al., 1985a; Starr, 1983; Travers & Stanton, 1984). The percentage with a positive attitude may however differ, depending on a number of factors. One factor is time spent at VDTs, which is confounded by type of job performed. In one field survey by Bolinder (1983), 62% of those working with VDTs less than 8 h/week were positive towards their work. The percentage reporting 'positive' decreased to 52% among those working more than 8 h/week, and to 28% among those working more than 20 h/week with VDTs. However, another study, cited by Dainoff (1982b), reported higher job satisfaction with increasing time spent at VDTs.

Job dissatisfaction was 70% among data-entry workers, compared to 28% among interactive communication-mode workers, in one study by Elias and coworkers (1982).

Consequences of the introduction of VDTs. With the present rapid introduction of VDTs in many workplaces, the majority of the present operators has not had too many year's experience working with VDTs. Data in some studies show differences in attitude according to number of years of VDT work, with the type of work presumably a strong confounder.

With the introduction of VDTs in office work, some investigators have suggested that a further 'polarization' of the work force into qualified and unqualified personel may occur. One example is secretaries, that may transform into 'administrative' and 'word-processing' secretaries (Warr, 1981; Westlander, 1984). This may have consequences for centralization of work, work measurements and social contacts (Warr, 1981). The increasing number of personal computers may, however, diminish such trends; for example, 'word-processing' secretaries may become less common.

Overall, several psychosocial changes have been recorded during the introductory phase of VDTs in offices (see Sell, 1984; Westlander, 1984). Involved in the etiology are such factors as 'novelty', 'need to practice', 'change in control of work', etc. These factors affected job satisfaction, job motivation, conflicts, qualifications, etc. Some changes recorded did, however, appear to be rather short-lived - concern with motivation/satisfaction being replaced by concern with monotony/turnover (Westlander, 1984). Westlander (1986) has presented some further study results on the effects of VDT introduction on three different offices. Work involving writing had changed considerably in one office, with the result that there was a reduced output of documents. This was, after analysis, assumed to be caused not by the introduction of VDT equipment per se, but by changes in organization during the VDT introduction phase.

The possibility of bias in reporting. In addition to possible
interactions with health effects, subjective psychosocial stress factors may
influence the self-reporting of various physical health effects. This is of
primary importance in conducting field or epidemiological studies - especially
if questionnaire responses are low. A brief discussion of bias is given when
discussing epidemiological studies of pregnancy (Section 5.3.7).

5.3 Health considerations of work on visual display terminals

5.3.1 Effects on the eyes and vision

In this section, the occurrence and the possible etiology of subjective
complaints of transient eye-related problems will be discussed, as well as the
possibility that permanent, pathological damage to the eyes may develop.

Comparison of occurrences of eye strain between different studies is
somewhat problematical, due to the varying definitions used. Eye strain can
be defined, based on specifications of a number of symptoms. As discussed
briefly below, the response will be considerably influenced by the specific
definition used.

One definition of the term asthenopia has been put forward by the US
National Research Council's Panel on Impact of Video Viewing on Vision of
Workers (1983). It refers to asthenopia as "any subjective visual symptoms or
distress resulting from the use of one's eyes". The symptoms of asthenopia
were then classified as: 1) visual (e.g. blurring); 2) ocular (eyes feel
tired, hot, uncomfortable or painful); 3) referral (e.g. headaches); and 4)
functional (behavioural). Other definitions of asthenopia may be found.

It is apparent that the term asthenopia, as defined here, includes a wider
spectrum of effects than ocular discomfort or eye strain. In the present text,
the term asthenopia (and eye discomfort) will be used, restricted to visual
and ocular (groups of) symptoms. Headache will be discussed on pp. 119-122,
and behavioural reaction problems on pp. 122-130. The terms 'eye strain' and
'visual complaints' will be used, when reference is made to a specific report,
where the term is explicitly or implicitly defined. In some studies, eye
strain does roughly correspond to the ocular group of symptoms of asthenopia.

5.3.1.1 <u>Asthenopia</u>

<u>Occurrence of eye discomfort among VDT-operators</u>. VDT-operators (as a group) have high incidences of asthenopia. Reported incidences from field studies vary, levels between 40-92% (at least occasional) to 10-40% (daily) have been reported. They were classified as both visual and ocular (Dainoff et al., 1981; Dainoff, 1982a; Elias et al., 1982; Grandjean, 1980; Gunnarsson & Söderberg, 1979; Gunnarsson & Söderberg, 1983; Kajiwara, 1984; Knave et al., 1985a; Mellner & Moberg, 1983). The incidence varied considerably due to a number of factors related both to the work situation (see below) and the study design.

Most studies report higher incidences of asthenopia in VDT-workers than in corresponding non-VDT workers (Belluci & Mauli, 1984; Bolinder, 1983; Canadian Labour Congress, 1982; Dainoff, 1982a; Frank, 1983; Ghingirelli, 1982; Kajiwara, 1984; Knave et al., 1985a; Läubli et al., 1981; Murray et al., 1981a; Nishiyama et al., 1984; Ong et al., 1981; Rey et al., 1982; Smith, M.J. et al., 1981). It should however be noted that often traditional office workers also report high incidences of asthenopia (Grandjean, 1980; Kajiwara, 1984; Knave et al., 1985a; Murray et al., 1981a; Starr, 1983; Turner, 1982).

In some studies (Gould & Grischkowsky, 1984; Lewis et al., 1982; Turner, 1982) no significant difference was found as to asthenopia. Sauter (1984) found that the use of VDTs <u>per se</u> was not predictive of eye strain, except that it did correlate with other factors that were predictive: e.g. display and workroom lighting problems. Starr (1984) found that asthenopia tended to be higher among VDT workers than controls, however, the differences were not statistically significant. The results of Howarth & Istance (1985) are discussed in some details below (p. 89).

Some of these complaints may still give rise to symptoms the next day (Läubli et al., 1981; Mellner & Moberg, 1983; Smith, 1982). Läubli and coworkers (1981) found that 40-45% of VDT workers reported visual impairments at the end of the day compared with 18-31% of non-VDT-workers, during watching television 11-19% compared with 7-14%, while reading 11-15% compared with 6-8%, when going to sleep 13-17% compared with 8-13%, next morning 2-8% compared with 0-2% and on Sundays 1-4% compared with 2-3%. The higher non-VDT

values were consistently found for typists. The visual symptoms
such as blurring often disappeared fairly rapidly after work (Smith, M.J.,
1982).

Occurrences of specific symptoms among VDT operators. The individual
symptoms noted differ between different field studies, but they can be
separated into two groups; in the first the eye being painful, irritated,
burning, red, tingling, having a gritty feeling, etc., all related to ocular
asthenopia symptoms; and in the second vision being blurred, double or
flickering, i.e. visual asthenopia symptoms (Bolinder, 1983; Canadian Labour
Congress, 1982; Elias et al., 1982; Frank, 1983; Grandjean, 1980; Läubli et
al., 1981; Rey et al., 1982; Starr, 1983). In Fig. 5, the occurrences of
some ocular symptoms in one investigation of office workers are shown,
separately for men and women.

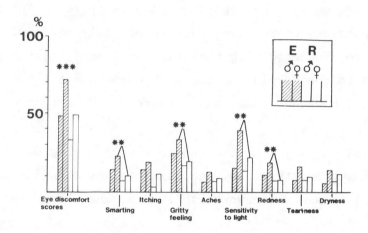

Fig. 5: Frequency of eye discomfort and the various eye symptoms in the
exposed (diagonally striped columns) and reference (unstriped columns) groups
distributed according to sex ($\male$ = men, $\female$ = women). The significance
indications refer to comparisons between the women in the exposed and
reference groups (** $p < 0.01$, *** $p < 0.001$). From Knave et al. (1985a).

In most studies, the ocular symptoms were more frequent than the visual
ones (Elias et al., 1982; Kajiwara, 1984; Läubli et al., 1981; Murray et al.,
1981b) but this was not always apparent (Canadian Labour Congress, 1982;
Starr, 1983). Turner (1982) found that no statistically significant
difference was seen as to asthenopia (total), however, a statistically
significant increase compared to non-VDT workers was seen in 'fatigue-like'
effects, for all VDT worker groups except 'creative'.

In a short note by Greenwald and coworkers (1983), a colour visual after-effect (McCullough effect) was described. Operators watching a display with green characters on a dark background did afterwards see a pink discoloration of white objects. The effect could last for a day or longer, but it was not considered permanent nor harmful. A prolonged complementary chromatopsia (30 min after cessation of work) was noted by Khan et al. (1984). Murray and colleagues (1981a) noted that 'change in colour vision' were reported more frequently among VDT- than among non-VDT workers. The occurrences varied considerably between workplaces though, from 8% in VDT workers compared to 5% in non-VDT workers at one site, to 90% compared to 63% in another.

5.3.1.2 Correlations between eye discomfort and other variables

The relationships between asthenopia and other VDT work characteristics are many. This discussion will be separated into two parts. The first, presented below, emphasizes confounding factors of field studies, while the next part will be more concerned with possible functional relationships specifically related to the display or the work environment. The distinctions between these two are, however, sometimes diffuse.

Male/female ratios and age. Women tend to report higher occurrences of visual or ocular symptoms than men, according to the Canadian Labour Congress Study (1982), Knave and coworkers (1985a), and Wallin and colleagues (1983).

Differences in reporting symptoms were not correlated with the age of the VDT operators according to the investigations of the Canadian Labour Congress, (1982), Knave and coworkers (1985a) or Mellner & Moberg, (1983). The higher incidence of asthenopia in persons aged 36-65 years compared to those aged 18-35, as found by Rey and coworkers (1982), was not statistically significant. In a later report, however, Meyer and colleagues (1985) did observe that subjects older than 40 years were consistently found in the group with more pronounced discomforts, but they did not complain as to lighting conditions. Younger subjects were found in this but also in other groups. Ong & Phoon (1986) found more frequent visual complaints among older (aged 31-45 years) than among younger (18-30 years) female VDT-operators, both groups doing data-entry work at the same site. The difference was statistically significant. Levy & Ramberg (1986) did not find any significant difference in eye-fatigue between younger and older women, but those authors noted that the frequencies may have been influenced by younger women doing more data-entry work.

Work categories. In principle, the type of work has a clear influence on the appearance of asthenopia.

Data-entry, data-acquisition and conversational-work operators generally tend to report high incidences (Canadian Labour Congress, 1982; Läubli et al., 1981; Sauter, 1984; Turner, 1982). Läubli and coworkers (1981), found conversational-mode VDT workers to have the highest occurrences of each investigated symptom, with data entry and traditional typists lower, and traditional office workers lowest. Knave and colleagues (1985a) found significant difference in reported eye strain between conversational VDT-operators and aquisition workers. A high frequency was found of 'eye fatigue' and 'painful eyes' among computer-assisted design-operators by Van der Heiden and coworkers (1984), comparable to those of data-entry operators, and higher than those experienced by traditional office workers.

Examining the persistence of the discomforts, however, the data-entry workers had more persistent occurrences according to Läubli and colleagues (1981). Furthermore, the Canadian Labour Congress study (1982), reported data-entry workers to have more ocular but less visual impairment (difficulty focusing) than conversational VDT workers.

Howarth and Istance (1985) compared four different groups, two working with VDTs and two with traditional office work. They reported that data-preparation workers (VDT) had a significant increase in discomforts during the workday on Mondays, a finding which was not observed on other days, nor for other groups. In comparison with data from other studies reported here, however, they also reported differences between groups as to discomforts reported at the end of the day. The data-preparation group reported higher occurrences compared to the other groups. Comparisons of word processors (VDT) and typists (non-VDT) did not reveal any differences in visual discomforts between these groups.

Duration of work and work breaks. The majority of studies indicated that
the occurrence of asthenopia increased with increasing working time at VDTs
(Canadian Labour Congress, 1982; Ghingirelli, 1982; Mellner & Moberg, 1983;
Murray et al., 1981a; Rey et al., 1982; Turner, 1982; Wallin et al., 1983),
usually with a 'break point' after four hours of work (Canadian Labour
Congress, 1982; Rey et al., 1982; Turner, 1982; Wallin et al., 1983). The
symptoms investigated included both ocular and visual symptoms.

In contradiction to these findings, some studies did not show any
correlation between work duration at VDT and asthenopia (Starr, 1984; Sauter,
1984). It should be noted that these studies, in contrast to many others,
included an analysis of the effects of other variables. Thus, it is
conceivable that the effects seen by many investigators are due more to the
type of job performed (and its corollaries) and the lighting problems than to
the working time per se. The results of Knave and coworkers (1985a), however,
indicate that work duration, especially the time looking at the screen, may be
a primary factor in determining asthenopia.

The duration of work without breaks has also been investigated. In the
study by Mellner and Moberg (1983) there was a significant positive
correlation between the duration of work without a break and the frequency of
symptom occurrence. Of those working less than 30 min without a break, 47%
complained of 'visual fatigue' compared with 66% of those working more than 30
min without a break.

Psychosocial aspects of work. Some studies have investigated the
correlation between subjective work evaluation and asthenopia. In the
Canadian Labour Congress study (1982), eye problems were more prominent in
workers who had less control, higher work pressure and high job
dissatisfaction. In further analysing a part of this material as to effects
of confounding variables, the relationship between visual discomforts and job
pressure was retained (Rowland, 1984). Worry showed a positive correlation
with asthenopia according to Wallin and colleagues (1983). An association
between job attitudes (work being hard, fast and with insufficient time to do
the job) and symptoms was indicated by A.B. Smith and coworkers (1982), but
the results were not retained in the predictive model analysis.

The regimentation of work and of work demands is an important factor as indicated by Sauter (1984) and M.J. Smith (1982). In a Bell Canada investigation, international operators showed more frequent eye strain symptoms (with a few exceptions) than did the local operators. Wilkins (1983), reviewing this investigation, suggested that the higher stress on the international operators might be a factor.

In another study by Knave and coworkers (1985a), no association between job attitudes and interest with eye discomfort symptoms was found.

The possible influence of visual disorders on VDT-related asthenopia. It has been suggested that preexisting visual disorders may influence the appearance of these symptoms in VDT operators (Campbell & Durdent, 1983). Thus, two uestions may be asked: 1) Do visual disorders influence the appearance of asthenopia? and 2) Can differences in preexisting visual disorder frequencies explain the differences found between VDT operators and controls as to asthenopia?

VDT operators who wear spectacles tend to report more eye troubles than VDT operators who do not (Böös et al., 1985; Läubli et al., 1981; Mellner & Moberg, 1983; Rubino et al., 1986; Sauter, 1984; Smith, M.J. 1982). This applies mainly to wearers of monofocal glasses (Böös et al., 1985, Sauter, 1984). It is possible that incorrect glasses and slight non-corrected astigmatism may be related to these findings, and also the increased reading distance to VDTs compared to 'normal reading' (Campbell & Durdent, 1983; Gunnarsson & Söderberg, 1983). This tendency of a correlation between complaints and use of glasses was also seen in the control groups (Läubli et al., 1981).

Some studies by Böös et al. (1985), and others cited in Dainoff (1982b), indicate that the asthenopia symptoms were not in general related to visual acuity defects, since optical correction had not alleviated the problems in the majority of workers seeking clinical help for their eye troubles. Furthermore, visual defects as regards visual acuity, accommodation, binocular vision, etc. were not significantly higher in VDT- than in non-VDT workers, although the incidence of asthenopia was higher (Böös et al., 1985; Nyman et al., 1985; Rey & Meyer, 1982). In older people a possible correlation was noted by Rey and coworkers (1982) between decreased visual acuity and increased visual complaints at VDTs.

In the study by Läubli et al. (1981) a positive correlation was seen between low visual acuity and impairments at VDTs, but not between uncorrected eye defects and complaints. Grignolo and colleagues (1984) found a relationship between subjective complaints with a score derived from a number of eye function tests; refraction, cover test, fusion, etc. In a later presentation of this study (Rubino et al., 1986) heterophoria was specifically correlated with eye discomforts. A similar result was found by Nyman and colleagues (1985), concerning exophorias and discomforts. Järvinen and Mäkitie (1986), however, did not notice any such correlation (see further p. 96 on heterophoria).

Irritated conjuctiva was seen more in VDT-workers with ocular asthenopia, but this was not seen in controls by Läubli and coworkers (1981). It was concluded by those authors that "work at VDTs may cause impairments in operators both with and without eye defects".

Correlation to musculoskeletal symptoms. In some studies (Hünting et al., 1981; Knave et al., 1985a; Läubli et al., 1981) the same operators who experienced musculoskeletal problems also indicated eye impairments. The authors suggested that this may be due to the more exacting conditions of work, producing a 'general fatigue', manifested as both musculoskeletal and visual problems. Such relationships were also found by Mellner and Moberg (1983) and by Sauter and coworkers (1983b).

However, the results reported by A.B. Smith and coworkers (1982) do indicate a more specific relationship, where bothersome lighting aspects of the VDT units would produce both asthenopia symptoms and a tendency of the operator to compensate for difficult viewing conditions - at the cost of musculoskeletal symptoms. In one study by Böös and colleagues (1985) a correlation was found between wearing of glasses and muscular discomfort.

5.3.1.3 <u>Studies on temporary changes in eye functions</u>

The occurrence of subjective eye discomforts has motivated the study of
visual and oculomotor functions in attempts to describe the reported
discomforts as symptoms of eye fatigue. According to the US National Research
Council (1983) temporary changes in oculomotor functions may be due to: 1) true
muscular fatigue; 2) adaptation of the sensory organs; 3) habituation of the
central nervous system; or 4) decline in motivation. Thus, in general,
relationships between subjective measures of fatigue (included in asthenopia)
and physiological functions have not been successfully established.

<u>Occurrence of changes in accommodation performance in VDT workers</u>.
Accommodation parameters studied are the near point of accommodation, the
focusing accuracy (accommodation point relative to specified test objects),
accommodation time (time taken to change accommodation from the near point to
the far point) and the position of the dark focus. Some fluctuations in
accommmodation (e.g. at the far point) have also been measured. Accommodation
in relation to specific screen parameters - flicker, blurr/sharpness and
contrasts - are discussed on pages 99-102.

<u>Studies of accommodation near point</u>. These studies have generally been
carried out with the use of an RAF near point ruler. The assumption is that
fatigue in the ciliary and oculomotor muscles would tend to limit the ability
to accommodate to near distances.

In a large field study by Nyman et al. (1985) of 505 workers (379 VDT
operators), no change in accommodation capacity was seen during the workday,
neither among VDT-operators nor among non-VDT workers. The study population
was stratified as to age. A similar negative finding was also reported by
Hedman and Briem (1984) in a study of 30 telecommunication operators. Both of
these studies showed a distinct increase of the near point distance with age.
Some changes in accommodation were noted between VDT operators with and without
eye discomfort by Järvinen and Mäkitie (1986), but only in the older age groups.

Changes in the near point during the workday were examined during 'normal'
and 'intensive' VDT work for three different groups (Gunnarsson & Söderberg,
1983). One younger group of 11, aged less than 35 years, showed a significant
increase in near point during intense work, while two other older groups failed

to show any such significant changes. This study was criticized by the US National Research Council (1983) on several points. The criticism pointed to the use of samples of opportunity, scant information on demographic and work environments, and absence of appropriate referent groups. Furthermore, no information on visual status was presented, and the techniques used were such that general fatigue and subject motivation could have been involved. No information on statistical analysis was presented.

Three experimental studies involving small study groups also indicated changes in near point during VDT work (Kumashiro, 1984; Kurimato et al., 1983) or VDT-like displays (Nishiyama et al., 1982). These latter experimental studies are related to very intense work rather different from normal VDT work as reported from the negative field studies.

Studies of focusing accuracy. In these studies, the difference in distances to the eyes' focus and the placement of the test object was measured by laser optometry. The assumption is that fatigue should be manifested as a tendency to focus in a more narrow range around the dark focus, and thus a discrepancy between the focus and the object may occur more frequently.

In one study (Hedman & Briem, 1984), there were differences in focusing accuracy mainly correlated with age, and also with job intensity. During more intensive work, an increase in accommodation deviation (measured in dioptres) during the workday was found in all age groups. It was concluded that VDT work per se did not influence the accommodation, but that workload and age did. Furthermore, in a related paper by Shahnavaz and Hedman (1984), accommodation changes were correlated with screen luminances and various contrasts - darker screens or higher contrasts (screen/surround, screen character/background) indicating larger accommodation changes (changes were most evident during night-shift).

In another study (Ostberg, 1980), changes in focusing accuracy were attributed by the author to VDT work. It is possible, again, that this may reflect differences in workload.

Studies of accommodation time. Changes in the time to shift accommodation from the far to the near point during VDT work have also been investigated in some small, experimental studies.

The time taken for accommodation from the far to the near point (and reverse), was higher in VDT work than in hard copy work (the differences were about 12 - 13 ms) (Mourant et al., 1981). Changes in accommodation time were also seen during VDT work in another study (Kurimato et al., 1983).

Studies of dark focus. A general increase in dark focus (measured in dioptres) was seen in all age groups during intense work, but not during normal work (Hedman & Briem, 1984), however, the usefulness of dark focus measurements in evaluating accommodative stress has been questioned (Taylor & MvVey, 1984).

Studies on small fluctuations of accommodation. Fluctuation in the ciliary muscle was measured by an infrared optometer by Yamamoto and coworkers (1986), and changes in the low-frequency component were examined. Four subjects worked at VDTs during a preset scheme, which included rest breaks. The highest activity was noted at 11h00 (before lunch) and smaller peaks noted again at 14h00 and 16h00. Some correlations were noted between accommodation fluctuations and rest breaks in combination with work pace, although the results could only be considered preliminary.

General comments on accommodation. The studies referred to differ considerably in many important respects; populations, work intensity, field studies versus experimental ones, parameters studied, etc. There is no overall consistency in these findings: studies on the near point generally fail to indicate any effect, while the two studies on accommodation time do, and varying results have been obtained from studies on other accommodation parameters.

It is possible that effects of VDT work, and differences between VDT work and hard copy work are primarily detectable during intense work loads, such being more readily attained during experimental set ups compared to normal work studied in field investigations. No correlation was found in an epidemiological study by A.B. Smith and coworkers (1982) between VDT-use (hours/day, years of VDT-use or 'current VDT-use') and accommodation changes. Furthermore, accommodation (near point) could not be correlated with eye discomforts or work duration according to Nyman and coworkers (1985) as well as Järvinen and Mäkitie (1986).

Vergence in VDT workers. Few results related to VDT work have been reported. Nyman et al. (1985) did not find any differences in convergence during the workday for VDT workers, nor any correlation with eye discomfort symptoms or work duration parameters. Gunnarsson & Söderberg (1979) found that the near point of convergence moved outwards 1-4 cm during a day's VDT work. This effect was increased during intense as compared to normal work routines. Hedman (1982), however, found no difference in the near point of convergence before work compared with after work, or between VDT- and non-VDT workers.

Some experimental results have also appeared. The divergence time was increased after a VDT task-period compared to before the period, and the vergence amplitude was decreased. No change in convergence time was seen (Iwasaki & Kurimoto, 1984).

Heterophoria. A high percentage (about 25%) of VDT operators working at screens with low contrasts were reported to have occasionally occurring exophorias. No operators at screens with high contrasts reported exophoria (Läubli et al., 1981). Lateral phoria changed during the working day, both for VDT-exposed and control groups. There was no significant difference between VDT and control groups however. Both inward and outward movements of the far vergence point were seen. Vertical phorias were not affected (Gould & Grischkowsky, 1984)

Increased exophoria in VDT workers compared to controls was found by Järvinen & Mäkitie (1986). Woo and coworkers (1986) reported a trend towards esophoria during VDT work, which according to them may be linked to some form of chromatic adaptation.

In contrast to these findings, neither Nyman and coworkers (1985) nor Dainoff and colleagues (1981) found any changes during the working day in any type of heterophoria. Both studies used fairly large study groups, 505 and 121 individuals, respectively. As already reported (p. 92) Nyman and coworkers (1985) did however find a relationship between exophoria and visual discomfort.

Changes in refraction and visual acuity. Temporary reduction in visual
acuity during VDT work has been reported by Haider and colleagues (1982): from
visus 1.1 to 0.8 for green characters, and from 1.1 to 0.9 for yellow
characters. Recovery took about 15 min. Such temporary changes were also seen
by Ehrlich (1986), Jaschinski-Kruza (1984) and Woo and coworkers (1986). Other
studies (Dainoff, 1982a; Gould & Grischkowsky, 1984; Nyman et al., 1985), found
no significant differences in refraction or visual acuity before and after work
in VDT operators. It should be noted that visual acuity or refraction in the
reviewed studies was measured by different methods: Landolt rings,
refractometer, contrast sensitivity, making comparison difficult. See a brief
discussion by Jaschinski-Kruza (1984). In the study cited by Ehrlich (1986),
the subjects worked at a near distance (0.6 mm characters at 20 cm distance)
which makes comparison with VDT work difficult.

Flicker sensitivity. A few studies have investigated changes in critical
flicker fusion (CFF), i.e. the highest frequency at which the subject detects
flicker, for a set luminance and phosphor type. These studies have generally
used various experimental set-ups to detect CFF.

In one such experimental set-up, one hour exposure to 30 or 60 Hz
oscillating luminances decreased the CFF (Nishiyama et al., 1982). In
concordance with this, a decrease in the CFF was also seen after 90 min VDT
work, in another experimental study by Kumashiro, (1984). In still another
study by Gould and Grischkowsky (1984), however, no change was seen.

Meyer and coworkers (1986), investigated the relationships between flicker
annoyance and refresh rates. For a fast phosphor, annoyance was observed by
50% of those tested at 67 Hz, while the critical refresh rate was 63 Hz for a
slow phosphor. The luminance was 50 cd/m^2, the illuminated screen extended
30° of vision. By varying also luminance, it was shown that a wide variety
in individual sensitivy exists; comfortable reading (at 70 cd/m^2) was
possible for the least sensitive subject at about 55 Hz, but only at 88 Hz for
the most sensitive subject.

Pupil constriction. Transient adaption glare may cause transient changes
in pupil size, as indicated by experimental studies. Alternatively viewing a
negative polarity screen and positive polarity documents may then possibly
cause overexposure of the retina (Cakir et al., 1980). Others have criticized

the experimental basis for this suggestion, (Campbell & Durdent, 1983; National Research Council, 1983), primarily by pointing out differences between the experimental conditions and conditions during VDT work. Zwahlen and Hartman, (1985) measured pupil diameter changes during VDT and non-VDT work on six operators, and found no major pupillary adjustments when transferring the glance from a negative polarity display to a document.

5.3.1.4 Probable causes of discomfort among VDT operators

The findings by Sauter (1984), that VDT work per se did not produce increased ocular discomfort is of considerable interest. The study does not suggest that VDT use is not associated with ocular discomfort, but rather that improved display and workroom lighting characteristics can alleviate the problems. There is general agreement on this point, see National Research Council (1983).

Definite causal relationships between specific display or workroom characteristics and asthenopia symptoms have seldom been established, however. It has been suggested that asthenopia complaints are related to workroom lighting, glare, dry air, screen or character brightness, readability, flicker, or reflections (See Canadian Labour Congress, 1982; Dainoff, 1982; De Groot & Kamphuis, 1983; Knave et al., 1985b; Läubli et al., 1981; Mellner & Moberg, 1983; Padmos & Pot, 1986; Sauter, 1984; Smith, A.B. et al., 1982; Stammerjohn et al., 1981; Turner, 1982; Wu et al., 1986).

Data from part of the cohort examined in the Canadian Labour Congress study (1982) have been analysed by Rowland (1984) for the effect of confounding variables. A relationship between discomfort and flicker was confirmed, while the other relationships put forward by the Canadian Labour Congress study (1982) were not, e.g. between discomforts and lighting or ambient air conditions (see above).

Some indications in the study by A.B. Smith and coworkers (1982) suggest that ocular asthenopia may be primarily associated with workplace lighting characteristics (glare, brightness of main lighting, shadows, etc.) and not display characteristics, while some visual asthenopia symptoms may be more related to the display characteristics.

It should be emphasized that many of these studies used the operators subjective evaluations as to both the presumed independent display or workroom characteristics and the dependent eye discomfort variables. In a few studies, objective measurements, display or workroom characteristics were made (Knave et al., 1985b; Läubli et al., 1981).

Time-dependent display characteristics. As indicated above, visible flicker may be related to visual system discomfort. Flicker sensitivity being higher in peripheral vision, it has been argued that VDTs may be more annoying when not looked at, but situated in the visual periphery (Isensee & Bennett, 1983).

Läubli and coworkers (1981) found that the degree of oscillation of single characters on VDT screens used for conversational-mode work correlated positively with ocular symptoms, but not with visual symptoms. These findings were supported by medical observations of red conjuctivae. In an experimental set up by Nishiyama and colleagues (1982), asthenopia symptoms were more prominent after 60 min exposure to 30 Hz refresh rate than to 60 Hz or stable text. The experiment used a chopper disc to simulate the oscillation of VDT screen characters.

A positive correlation between the degree of annoyance by flicker and the degree of complaints of asthenopia was found by Stammerjohn and coworkers (1981), both for professional and for clerical VDT workers. Similar findings were made by the Canadian Labour Congress (1982). Flicker appears to affect the low frequency fluctuation of accommodation, according to Iwasaki and Kurimoto (1986).

Structure related display characteristics. Difficulties with character solution, distortions and readability are intimately linked with job task performance.

A significant correlation between annoyance as to low readability and high occurrence of asthenopia was found by M.J. Smith and coworkers (1982), but only for professional and not for clerical workers. The results were not subjected to multiregression analysis to account for the effects of other variables, and there are considerable problems of interpretation, as readability could be linked to glare, brightness, etc. (Stammerjohn et al., 1981). Focusing defects and blurred characters have been linked with asthenopia in the Canadian Labour Congress study (1982); and in the study by Turner (1982).

Luminance related display characteristics. Reported brightness of screen character has been associated with asthenopia (Smith, A.B. et al., 1982; Stammerjohn et al., 1981). In the second study, this effect was noted only for professional workers. These results were not analysed for potential confounding factors. In a large field study by Knave and coworkers (1985b), an increased difference between measured screen and manuscript luminance was associated with increased occurrence of eye discomfort (see Fig. 6).

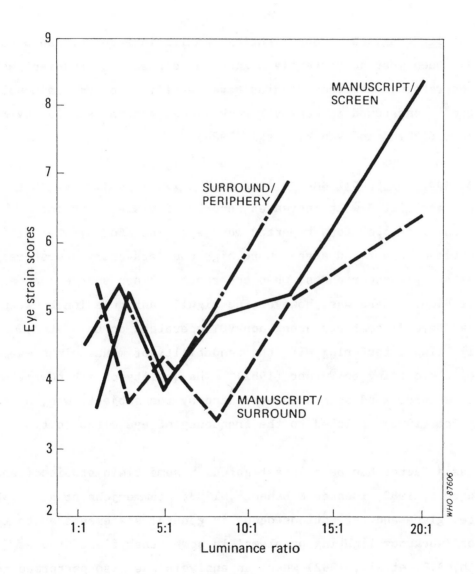

Fig. 6: Relationship between the luminance ratios and eye discomfort for the women in the exposed group. (surround = close surroundings.) From Knave et al. (1985b).

Shahnavaz and Hedman (1984) noted increased changes in accommodation with decreasing screen luminance. Low frequency accommodation fluctuation was influenced by contrast and peripheral luminance, according to Corno and Denieul (1986). The latter authors suggested that positive polarity in this respect is "sometimes more favourable than negative polarity". As stated previously, however, there are problems in relating changes in accommodation to subjective symptoms.

Workroom lighting. Workroom lighting and its interrelationship to the display have been most consistently suggested as possible causes of asthenopia among VDT operators. Numerous studies have testified to the inadequate lighting conditions found in many VDT-workplaces, see the studies by Murray and coworkers (1981a) and Von Kiparski (1984).

In the report by Läubli and colleagues (1981), it was noted that a high contrast was associated with increased reports of visual problems. Conversational-mode operators reported more eye discomforts, when differences between source document and screen were high and data-entry operators had more frequent asthenopia occurrences, when contrasts between source documents and tables were high. There was, however, no significant relation between contrasts and eye discomforts among non-VDT operators on this study. Low workroom lighting interfering with the readability of manuscripts was related to asthenopia according to Turner (1982). The quality of a handwritten manuscript, whether good or bad as evaluated by the subject, was, according to Padmos and Pot (1986), related to the frequency of eye discomfort.

Glare as a factor has been investigated in some field studies (Canadian Labour Congress, 1982; Isensee & Bennett, 1983; Stammerjohn et al., 1981). Furthermore, glare and reflections occur in general statements as to the presence of 'workroom lighting problems' in some other field studies (Sauter, 1984; Smith, A.B. et al., 1982) where an analysis was also performed to control for potential confounding factors.

A correlation between the occurrence of reflections and the occurrence of asthenopia has been found in some field studies (Dainoff, 1982; Mellner & Moberg, 1983), but not in others (Läubli et al., 1981).

Workroom environment. In a study by Rey and coworkers (1982) a reduced blink rate occurred due to: a) the duration of a difficult visual task; b) general low illumination levels (where the screen was surrounded by darkness); and c) the eye being myopic. However, higher blink rates have also been found among VDT users compared to non-VDT controls (Gould & Grischkowsky, 1984; Mourant et al., 1981).

As discussed in Campbell & Durdent (1983), a reduced blink rate could cause a drying effect and mild anoxia of the corneal epithelium. The problem would then be aggravated by low air humidity. An association between dry air and the occurrence of asthenopia has been suggested by the findings of the Canadian Labour Congress (1982). However, when a subcohort from this study was analysed by Rowland (1984) to check for confounding factors, the suggested association disappeared. Furthermore, Knave and coworkers (1985b) found no association between asthenopia and room humidity.

5.3.1.5 Pathological changes in the eyes

The possibility of permanent eye damage due to VDT work has been suggested by Zaret (1984) and Kajiwara (1984). Considerable debate has been aimed at the question of cataracts, but acquired myopia has also figured in discussions of the effect of VDTs.

Cataracts among VDT operators. Cataracts are the formation of opacities in the eye lenses, which may (if sufficiently dense) lead to impairment and loss of vision. Small opacities occur in most old people's eyes, and are one of the most frequent reasons for loss of visual acuity. Cataracts are due to a number of factors, some of which (radiation) have been considered in the context of VDTs. The development of cataracts after ionizing radiation is a prolonged process, with a latent period of months to years.

Cataracts may be defined according to appearance (nuclear, cortical etc.) and to severity. In the present context, cataracts are described as 'all lens opacities' or as 'opacities connected with a decrease in visual acuity'. The exact definition may differ between different ophthalmologists, which has caused some problems of interpretations, see Böös and colleagues (1985). Some studies, Canadian Labour Congress (1982) and Frank (1983) apparently only

reported cataracts that interfered with vision, but did not explicitly state
the decrease in visual acuity considered in the diagnosis, whereas other
studies (Böös et al., 1985; Smith, A.B. et al. 1982) included all opacities
and also classified visual acuity decrease in specified subgroups.

In 1977, two cases of cataract in New York were diagnosed by their
ophthalmologists as incipient radiant energy cataracts. These diagnoses were
confirmed by another expert, whose diagnoses read: "Bilateral incipient
radiant energy cataracts and early macular retinopathy of the left eye" (case
1) and "Immature radiant energy cataract of the right eye and incipient
radiant energy cataract of the left eye" (case 2) (Zaret, 1980).

Both these men (aged 29 and 34 years) worked as copy editors at the New
York Times, and both had within the last few years been introduced to VDT work.
For neither of them could a reasonable and established work environmental
factor causing the injury be found, although the possibility of a pre-existing
congenital defect was suggested by the consulting ophthalmologist of the
newspaper. This latter suggestion was disputed by Zaret (1980).

Since then, Zaret (1980) has made similar diagnoses in at least eight
other cases all working with CRT equipment. In the majority of these ten
cases, the cataracts were described as 'capsular opacification at the
posterior surface of the lens' by Zaret, (1980; 1984). The US National
Research Council's Panel on Impact of Video Viewing on Vision of Workers
(1983), however, expressed serious doubts about the validity of a number of
these diagnoses and stated that "the panel found such conclusions unwarranted."

Epidemiological studies on the possibilities of a VDT/cataract
association. Four epidemiological studies have been performed concerning the
possibility of increased cataract formation among VDT operators, see Table 2.

Table 2. Performed epidemiological studies on cataracts among VDT operators

Study and reference	Method	Increase in lens opacities	
		All lens opacities	Associated with decrease in visual acuity
Baltimore Sun (Smith, A.B. et al., 1982)	Exam.	No	No
Newspaper Guild (Frank, 1983)	Quest.	-	Not eval. [a]
Canadian Labour Congress, 1982	Quest.	-	No [b]
NBOSH (Böös et et al., 1985)	Exam. [c]	No [d]	No [d]

Exam. = diagnosis by ophthalmological examination, Quest. = information received via questionnaire, diagnosis thus by different physicians and subject to possible selection bias by respondents. No = no significant increase in cataract occurrence in VDT operators compared to controls. Not eval. = outcome could not be evaluated, according to the author.

[a] Incomplete information in Frank (1983); 16 of 18 cataracts were found among VDT operators (that comprised 74% of the material), but "many had developed prior to exposure of these individuals to VDTs".

[b] Stratified as to age.

[c] Three physicians involved, each examined different groups; no random assignment, they were not blind to exposed/control status of examinee.

[d] No statistically significant (borderline for all opacities) increase among VDT compared to controls was noted, considerable differences between results of the different ophthalmologists were however noted - one ophthalmologist found most cataracts in controls, and two, most among VDT operators.

In the Baltimore Sun Study (Smith, A.B. et al., 1982), the incidence of all lens opacities was 27.1% among VDT users, and 33.2% among non-VDT users. Some 1.4 - 1.5% of both groups had sufficient cataract formation to reduce visual acuity to at least 20/25. The study encompassed 283 newspaper office workers.

In a second study (Newspaper Guild) of 1047 workers (Frank, 1983), the VDT-users reported 2% cataracts, while the non-VDT users had 0.7% cataracts, based on questionnaire report data, thus presumably including only 'opacities interfering with vision'. The report mentions also cases of pre-cataract conditions, but gives no details. Of these 16 cases, data were incomplete as to years of present employment or age of cataract manifestation; six occurred within "the previous five-year period". A cluster of cases in St Louis (ten cases) was also noted.

In a survey made by the Canadian Labour Congress (1982) the frequency of cataracts were: 1) for people under 45 years of age; 1.1% (VDT operators), 0.9% (non-VDT) versus 1% 'expected'; 2) for people over 45 years of age, 3.6% (VDT operators), 4.6% (non-VDT) versus 4% 'expected'.

In an ophthalmological study of 505 office workers in Stockholm (Böös et al., 1985), the percentage of all lens opacities were 8% (VDT operators) versus 3,5% (controls) and for pathological opacities 2.6% (VDT operators) versus 0.8 % (controls). These differences were not statistically significant. There were however major differences in the results from the three ophthalmologists who examined subjects from different workplaces (see notes in Table 2). The authors considered that the results did not point to VDT work as a factor in cataract formation. Nevertheless, the somewhat ambiguous data justify further follow-up of these examinees, and this is planned for 1987 - five years after the previous examinations.

Some epidemiological shortcomings should be noted. Both the Canadian Labour Congress study (1982) and the study by Frank (1983) were limited to subjective responses on questionnaires. In the study by Böös and colleagues (1985) ophthalmological examinations were performed, but since large differences were noted between ophthalmologists, and since the examinees were

not randomly assigned to these ophthalmologists, this study also has
methodological problems, as pointed out by the authors. The study by Frank
(1983) had a low response rate (40%) compared to 81% for the Canadian Labour
Congress study (1982). In the study by A.B. Smith and coworkers (1982) 50% of
the cohort were examined, compared to 86% in the study by Böös and colleagues
(1985).

Suggested VDT factors involved in cataractogenesis. The only known
relevant VDT-dependent factor for cataractogenesis is electromagnetic
radiation. Four regions of the electromagnetic spectrum are considered
(possibly) cataractogenic: ionizing, UV-A, infrared and microwave radiation,
all dependent on a sufficient dose. For all of these regions, the levels now
known to produce cataracts are orders of magnitude higher than those possibly
emitted from VDTs (Lerman, 1980; Pitts et al., 1980; WHO, 1979).

Zaret (1980) suggested that UV radiation from VDT might produce
cataracts. However, in the study reported by Knave and coworkers (1985b) and
by Böös and colleagues (1985), it was found that the total exposure to UV-A in
offices was significantly lower for VDT-workstations (approximately 4
$\mu W/cm^2$) than for non-VDT-workstations (approx. 13 $\mu W/cm^2$) and strongly
correlated with the general illumination (presumably from windows).
Furthermore the measured UV-A levels were not correlated with the appearance
of lens opacities.

The presented data show that radiation emission from VDTs cannot be
considered as a credible cause of cataract formation in VDT operators.

Myopia development due to VDT work. A Japanese survey by Kajiwara (1984)
of 1580 VDT operators and 125 controls has suggested that VDT work may lead to
nearsightedness, since the number of people who were prescribed corrective
glasses during a one year period was higher than normal; 37% of the VDT
operators reported deteriorating eyesight, compared to 26% in controls.
Specific details critical to the evaluation of this suggestion are not
presented in the report.

Another study by Frank (1983) revealed no significant differences in the
number of eyeglass prescription changes between VDT users and nonusers, but,

as no details were given on the type of eyeglasses, and, in view of the low response rate in this study, evaluation of the study is difficult.

Both these studies use occurrences of prescriptions as an indicator of a possible VDT-specific effect. The use of such an indicator is also questionable, since it is possible, as discussed by Wilkins (1983), that the visual effort required when working with VDTs is such that the operators also tend to correct existing minor visual impairments, while similar impairments among persons in similar, non-VDT jobs may be ignored or even go undetected.

In the study by Böös and colleagues (1985) examinations of 379 VDT operators and 125 controls did not reveal any differences between VDT operators and controls as to spherical refraction, measured by a refractometer or ascertained by routine examinations by ophthalmologists. The data were stratified as to age.

Other possible permanent eye damage investigated. A number of other indicators of permanent eye damage have been routinely investigated in the questionnaires and the ophthalmological examinations of some epidemiological studies, without the detection of differences between VDT-exposed and controls. Disorders investigated include glaucoma, maculopathy, iris inflammation, etc., but, there are at present no indications that VDT-exposure may lead to increased incidence of these manifestations (Frank, 1983; Grignolo et al., 1986; Smith, A.B. et al., 1982).

It should however be noted, that few epidemiological studies have thus far studied in detail the possibilities of chronic visual disturbances due to VDT work (Smith, M.J. 1982). Furthermore, the possibility of relationships between pre-existing disorders and VDT-caused visual discomfort has not been elucidated.

5.3.2 Musculoskeletal discomforts

Several studies have investigated the occurrence of musculoskeletal discomfort among VDT operators. These symptoms may be of various types (pain, stiffness, fatigue or tiredness, cramps, numbness, tremor, etc.), occur at various locations in the body (neck, shoulder, arms, etc.) and occur with varying frequency for each operator affected (daily, occasionally, seldom or never).

Most are field studies, based on subjective reports on muscular discomfort. These questionnaires were in some studies supplemented by medical observations of painful pressure points, electromyography recordings or posture measurements. Some, but not all, field studies used control groups. Job task classification were made in some studies. Confounding factors (notably male/female ratios) have been checked for only in a few studies.

5.3.2.1 Occurrence of musculoskeletal symptoms

Musculoskeletal discomforts are probably the most commonly reported complaint in most offices. This appears true also of offices using VDTs. In Sweden, most reports to the official inquiry register for suspected occupational diseases in work with visual display terminals concerned musculoskeletal discomforts (NBOSH, 1985b). The issue at hand is whether work with VDTs introduces an increased frequency of complaints, and whether there is a unique character of these complaints, due to display and workstation design, or to changes in the performed jobs.

When comparing musculoskeletal complaints from VDT operators with appropriate controls, the results have been varied. One study testifies to the higher occurrences of musculoskeletal problems among VDT operators (Frank, 1983), while most have failed to find significant or consistent higher occurrences (Bolinder, 1983; Canadian Labour Congress, 1982; Gould & Grischkowsky, 1984; Knave et al., 1985a; Löfgren, 1985; Sauter et al., 1983b). In the report by Murray and coworkers (1981b), an increase in musculoskeletal complaints during VDT work was seen in one of three worksites examined (see discussion on sex distribution below). In the report by A.B. Smith and coworkers (1982), VDT users were found to suffer greater musculoskeletal discomfort than non-VDT users, but this result did not survive analysis for confounding factors.

In the research report by Murray and coworkers (1981b), three workplaces were examined, in two of which results were reported from subjects being asked both whether a specific symptom 'has occurred' and whether the symptom

'occurred frequently or constantly'. For both VDT- and non-VDT users, the
latter responses were between 10% and 50% of the former. A more detailed
analysis (made by the reviewer) shows that in these two sites (each comprising
some 100-150 subjects), there was a tendency of VDT operators to state that
their reported symptoms were 'frequent or constant' to a higher degree than
the controls. Similar observations were made in Bolinder (1983) where VDT
operators tended to report their problems as more serious than did controls.
Another investigation, cited in a paper by Grandjean (1980) however, revealed
no such differences.

Musculoskeletal symptoms in various body locations. More definite
differences between different types of jobs (including both VDT and non-VDT
jobs) were seen when specific complaint locations were examined.

In one study by Hünting and coworkers (1981), data-entry workers (VDT) and
typists (non-VDT) had more complaints in the neck and shoulder regions than
conversational-mode workers (VDT) or traditional office workers (non-VDT).
These subjective symptoms were verified by medical examination, and were also
manifested as painfully limited head mobility. A higher incidence of primarily
neck and shoulder complaints among some types of VDT jobs compared to some non-
VDT jobs have also been seen in a number of other studies (Canadian Labour
Congress, 1982; Frank, 1983; Grieco et al., 1982; Nishiyama et al., 1984).
Kemmlert and colleagues (1986), however, did not find more frequent neck and
shoulder problem among VDT operators compared to other office workers, but
indicated that "traditional office machinery causes just as many physical
effects".

Data-entry workers (VDT), conversational-mode workers (VDT) and typist
(non-VDT) complained more than traditional office workers (non-VDT) of back
pain (Hünting et al., 1981).

Data-entry workers (VDT) had more arm complaints than had conversational-mode workers (VDT) and typists (non-VDT), who in turn had more complaints than traditional office workers (non-VDT). Pain in isometric contractions of the forearm increased in the order traditional office worker - conversational-mode workers - typists - data-entry workers. Upper leg problems were reported primarily by data-entry workers (VDT), followed by traditional office workers (non-VDT) (Hünting et al., 1981).

An increased frequency of more centrally localized discomforts, e.g. in the shoulders and back among VDT operators compared to controls, were also seen by Knave and coworkers (1985a), as indicated in Figure 7. (Note that these data concern "symptom points", where also intensity of discomforts is considered.) In the study by Löfgren (1985), neck, shoulder and back problems were more frequent than peripheral problems, but there were fairly small differences between VDT operators and controls. The author suggests that this may reflect an 'optimal workload'.

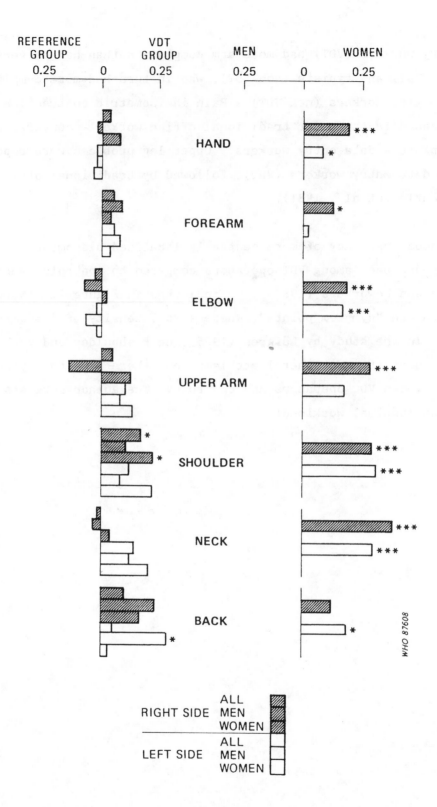

Fig. 7: Location of musculoskeletal complaints. Score differences between the entire exposed (VDT) and reference groups and between the men and the women of the two groups (* p < 0.05, *** p < 0.001). From Knave et al. (1985a).

5.3.2.2   Correlations between musculoskeletal symptoms and other variables

Sex and age of the operator. The sex of the operator appears to have a strong influence on the reporting of musculoskeletal problems. In the research report by Murray and coworkers (1981b) the average reporting symptom frequency (14 questions) was apparently related to the sex of the VDT operator. In the investigation by Knave and colleagues (1985a) women had more muscle discomfort complaints than men, both as to 'any localization' and as to all specific localizations. Kemmlert and coworkers (1986) also reported a higher incidence of neck and shoulder complaints among women than among men in office work.

In Wallin et al. (1983), a number of possible confounders related to work periods, job types, organization etc., were shown to be different between men and women of the study. Unfortunately, few studies have been conducted where both sex (male/female) and various jobs characteristics have been analysed as to their impact on the reported discomfort. Sauter and coworkers (1983a) in performing such an analysis, did not find any associations with VDT per se, but did find associations with other variables, such as VDT workstation design.

In the study by Kemmlert and coworkers (1986), neck and shoulder troubles were found more frequently among older subjects. Ong & Phoon (1986) also found increased discomforts among older subjects (all women), but suggested that increased household work among the older women might also have contributed. (See previous discussion on pp. 73-74).

Work categories. As indicated above, the type of job has a strong influence on the reported musculoskeletal complaints. In general, data-entry workers often have a higher incidence of pain reported in specific locations, as compared both to non-VDT-workers (Canadian Labour Congress, 1982; Sauter, 1984; Hünting et al., 1981) and to other VDT jobs (Canadian Labour Congress, 1982; Elias et al., 1982; Hünting et al., 1981; Mellner & Moberg, 1983). Interactive communication resulted in more muscle pain than data acquisition according to Knave and coworkers (1985a).

Other types of work result in more varied responses between VDT- and non-VDT workers. Clerical VDT workers reported more complaints than their

non-VDT counterparts, while professional VDT- or telephone VDT operators did
not (Canadian Labour Congress, 1982). In one Canadian study, a considerable
difference in back muscle pain was found between international and local
telephone operators (both using VDTs): the reported incidences were 48%
compared with 24% [cited from Wilkins (1983), where this was suggested to be a
result of stress].

   Duration of work. A higher incidence of neck, shoulder or back complaints
is found with the increasing time spent at the VDT (Canadian Labour Congress,
1982; Gould & Grischkowsky, 1984; Mellner & Moberg, 1983; Sauter, 1984; Wallin
et al., 1983; Wilkins, 1983). The incidence of pain in the arms, hands or
legs has been found to be associated with increasing time spent at the VDT by
Wallin and coworkers (1983), but not by A.B. Smith and coworkers (1982). The
study population by Wallin and coworkers (1983) was investigated in a
follow-up study three years later (Wright, 1986). VDT operators with limited
VDT work experienced a decrease in musculoskeletal symptoms, while those of
extensive users had remained constant. Those reporting muscle discomforts had
longer working times (during one test day, but not on another), and times
spent looking at the screen than had those without complaints according to
Knave and colleagues (1985a). However, when multivariate analysis was
performed to check for the influence of different job types, the association
with working time disappeared in the the study by Sauter and coworkers
(1983a), and also in a subgroup of the Canadian Labour Congress study, as
reported by Rowland (1984).

   The increase in reported pain was found to be a fairly monotonous function
of the working hours, both in field studies (Canadian Labour Congress, 1982;
Wallin et al., 1983) and in an experimental study (Gould & Grischkowsky,
1984). A survey by Evans (1986), suggested that "often" painful/stiff neck or
shoulder increased at 5 h VDT work per day or more. (This study does,
however, suffer from potential selection bias, since the option of responding
to the questionnaire was open to readers of a magazine).

   The incidence of reported pain was significantly and positively correlated
with the length of the work periods (in the range 30 min - 2 h) (Mellner &
Moberg, 1983). Relief was noted during the lunch break (Gould & Grischkowsky,
1984). In a small study of six VDT word-processor operators, electromyography

measurements on the shoulder/neck trapezius muscles were made. Static work
was higher than recommended. A negative relationship between static work and
frequent (self-determined) short work breaks was seen, but not with a fixed or
predetermined pattern of short pauses (Hagberg et al., 1985).

Subjective evaluation of work. Pain and stiffness in the extremities were
not significantly associated with job-attitude variables, while pain and
stiffness in axial musculature were, especially with 'job being hard, fast,
with little time to do it'. These findings were however not verified by a
predictive model (Smith, A.B. et al., 1982).

Another study, which did not include an analysis to investigate potential
confounders, indicated a higher incidence of reported musculoskeletal pain
when: 1) the job was controlled by the system, not the user, 2) job pressure
was high, 3) job satisfaction was low (Canadian Labour Congress, 1982). The
relationship between pain and job pressure was retained by a "controlled"
analysis performed by Rowland (1984). Job demands was associated with
musculoskeletal pain according to Sauter and coworkers (1983a). In the
investigation by Knave and colleagues (1985a), no correlation was noted with
interest or attitude towards work.

Relation to display, illumination and eye strain. Pain and stiffness in
the shoulders, neck and back appear to be correlated also with visual aspects
of VDT work - such as bothersome lighting, glare and flicker. These findings
were supported by a model predictive analysis, but not by the study of a
second group of VDT/non-VDT workers in the same study (Smith, A.B. et al.,
1982). In some other studies (Knave et al., 1985b; Mellner & Moberg, 1983), a
positive correlation was noted between the occurrence of eye strain and
musculoskeletal complaints.

Wearing of glasses. It has been suggested that those presbyopes who lean
their heads back in order to use the lower part of their bifocal glasses may
be at a greater risk of developing muscle pain. Wearers of bifocal glasses
showed a slight (nonsignificant) tendency to increased muscle discomfort,
especially in the neck according to Böös and colleagues (1985). Prior to this
investigation, all examinees had been tested as to presbyope additions, and
given prescription for special glasses if such were required. It can thus be

assumed that many subjects had correct presbyope additions for the distance
involved at the time of this investigation. A.B. Smith and coworkers (1984)
found that wearers of bi- or multifocal glasses had lower incidences of pain
and aches in the axial musculature. This association was not, however,
verified by subsequent analysis of the data. It appears, that to evaluate the
importance of bifocal glasses, a measure of the actual presbyope addition
should be included. Thus far, this has not been the case. The wearing of
distance glasses, appears to be associated with increased muscle discomforts,
as found by Böös and colleagues (1985), and by Sauter and coworkers (1983a)
for musculoskeletal postural problems. According to Sandell and coworkers
(1986), head and neck movements tended to be greater with ordinary bifocals
than with those specified for VDT use.

5.3.2.3 <u>Etiology of the observed musculoskeletal complaints</u>

In principle, musculoskeletal problems among VDT users have been discussed
in connection with three general factors: first, repetetitive motions due to
keyboard typing which are briefly discussed under the heading of "permanent
damage", on pages 118-119; second, incorrect posture; and third,
immobilization. The last two are discussed below.

The various elements of the workstation may impose demands for viewing
distances etc., which are presumably met at the cost of postural problems.
This may be especially taxing when glare or reflections occur, causing severe
restraints as to optimal viewing posture.

The problems may be due both to incorrect posture (wrong ulnar deviation
of hand, excessive bending of the neck, changes in the lumbar region when
sitting - due both to chair characteristics and leg room, wrong elbow angle,
etc.), to static work (due to the absence of wrist or back support) and
immobilization (Hagberg et al., 1985; Hünting et al., 1981; Mellner & Moberg,
1983; National Research Council, 1983).

<u>Comparison with preferred settings</u>. In one field study by Hünting et al.
(1981) correlations were found between: 1) hand and arm pain and keyboard
height (above some 7-8 cm); 2) pains and excessive ulnar abduction (more than
20°); 3) absence of support for the arms and pains in the neck, shoulder and

arms and 4) increased head inclination and turning, with pains in the neck and shoulders. These findings correlate well with the general remarks made above and with the standards developed. A decrease in table height was associated with increased shoulder, neck and arm pain, but this was attributed to the absence of document holders, not the table height per se.

Similar confirmation has also been presented by Sauter (1984), where chair comfort and workstation configuration were found to be predictors of musculoskeletal pain. In specific situations, musculoskeletal strain increased with increasing viewing angle and was alleviated by the presence of a detached keyboard (this was not subject to multivariate analysis). In another field study by Murray et al. (1981b) excessive keyboard height above the floor or chair and excessive viewing angles were suggested to be associated with the occurrence of musculoskeletal problems. Due to the potential strong confounding influence of varying male/female ratios, no analysis is possible.

Correlations between bad postural workplace items (whether conforming to standard or not) and muscular complaints were noted also by Padmos & Pot (1986). As discussed elsewhere (pp. 67-68), suggested standard positions may not be fully applicable to VDT situations. Mandal (1986) indicated that people had less backache when sitting somewhat higher than advised by existing standards. For data-entry workers, this increased seating height was 7 cm above the recommended standard (CEN).

Sedentary work. Experience from space programmes, as well as with long-term hospital patients, has indicated that extreme physical inactivity may cause a variety of problems: physical deconditioning, decreased orthostatic tolerance, water and electrolyte disturbances, weight loss, bone demineralization and glucose intolerance. The extent to which such physiological effects may appear during moderate inactivity is still unknown (see review by Kilbom [1986]). Winkel (1986) has presented data on adverse effects of leg inactivity on foot and lower leg swelling, and suggests that a biphasic curve may exist for discomfort - this being higher both during low and high activity compared to moderate activity (such as combination of sitting, walking and standing).

A relation between certain stress and mood indicators and postural discomfort was noted by Zeier and coworkers (1986). The authors argue that this calls for programmes to "generate active behaviour instead of avoidance behaviour", in an attempt to avoid negative reinforcement of symptoms. It is also arguable that adverse stress or mood situations, in addition to functioning as negative reinforcements of experienced symptoms (as suggested above), may also prolong physical immobility and thus pain.

5.3.2.4 Repetitive motions and possible permanent damage

The existence of a cumulative trauma problem has been discussed for a variety of jobs, among both blue collar and white collar workers. Among the latter, keyboard operators have received considerable attention (Fergusson, 1984; Commonwealth Department of Health, 1985; National Occupational Health and Safety Commission, 1985). For VDT operators, Läubli (1986) noted a relationship between a high number of daily keystrokes and pain in the arms. This was suggested to be attributed to the rapid key speeds possible on modern keyboards, and the low force necessary, which have eliminated the need to involve the forearms. Thus, recommendations for an upright trunk and freely movable horizontal forearms may no longer be valid. A split keyboard may be more beneficial than the present traditional, one-piece keyboard. A case report of wrist trauma in a VDT operator has been described by Sauter and coworkers (1986b).

There is, however, considerable confusion as to terminology in this respect, including specific diagnostic terms such as carpal tunnel syndrome and tendonitis and general terms such as repetitive strain injury (RSI) or "teno" (derived from tenosynovitis) (Fergusson, 1984; Arndt, 1983).

Concern has been raised as to the possibility that organic injury may occur due to repeated stress in VDT work. This has been largely based on discussion of repetitive strain injury (RSI) in Australia, and the reported occurrences of such cases among VDT operators (Commonwealth Department of Health, 1985). However, the term RSI, as used in that report, includes the discomfort symptoms already described in the present section. The report of the Task Force on Repetition Strain Injury (Commonwealth Department of Health, 1985) does point out that there is disagreement as to whether RSI should be considered as a "physical and/or emotional stress leading to physical tension which results in organic injury (which may or may not be identifiable)" or a "physical and/or emotional stress being 'converted' to be expressed as a physical symptom in the form of real pain, but in the absence of organic injury". Rowe and coworkers (1986) have also commented on this problem in their reported study from Sydney and have suggested that RSI should probably be renamed "muscular fatigue related to working conditions".

Sauter and coworkers (1986a) examined four cases of chronic neck-shoulder discomfort in VDT workers, and noted that although the subjects experienced considerable discomfort, few objective indications of pathological effects could be seen. In three of these cases, there was little progression, and two cases improved considerably with changed working conditions. Although the findings can only be considered suggestive, the authors note that these cases do not support the suggestion of neurological or skeletal injury due to VDT work.

Evaluation of the suggestion that VDT operators may be at risk of musculoskeletal injury is not possible, based on the reviewed literature. The use of precise definitions of the operators' conditions is needed.

However, the discomfort experienced by many VDT operators should be taken seriously in terms of prevention and treatment regardless of our present inability to find a link between discomfort and organic injury or permanent damage in VDT operators.

5.3.3 Headache

Headache is considered a secondary symptom of asthenopia, but may also be related to stress disorders or to muscular discomfort. Due to the uncertain etiology, headache is considered separately in this chapter.

The occurrence of headaches among VDT operators. The percentage of VDT operators and controls complaining of headaches varies considerably between different studies, conceivably due both to different working situations and to the design of the field study questionnaires, as well as the ambiguity concerning the definition of headache. The incidences reported for both groups vary between 11% and 89% (Canadian Labour Congress,1982; Dainoff et al., 1981; Knave et al., 1985a, Lewis et al., 1982; Murray et al., 1981b; Smith, M.J. 1982; Starr, 1983; Sauter, 1983; Travers & Stanton, 1984; Wilkins, 1983).

Some field surveys have found a significant increase in reported headaches among VDT operators compared to controls (Canadian Labour Congress, 1982; Frank, 1983; Smith, A.B. et al., 1982), while other studies have failed to do so (Bolinder, 1983; Knave et al., 1985a; Lewis et al., 1982; Murray et al., 1981b; Smith, M.J. 1982; Starr et al. 1982; Wallin et al., 1983).

Different headache symptoms. Frontal headache occurred more among VDT operators than among controls (Frank, 1983). In the work by Ghingirelli (1982), 27% of VDT operators complained of frontal headaches not related to previous medical history.

In the report of A.B. Smith and coworkers (1982) 17 different headache descriptions were investigated in relation to a number of VDT work-descriptors. Details from the statistical analysis; these are shown in Table 3. When testing the significant results on a second group (with different job types), only headache associated with work was retained. The remaining 12 headache variants were not associated with VDT work-descriptors. See Table 3 for some examples, and A.B. Smith and coworkers (1982) for a full description.

Table 3. Different headache description and their relation with VDT work parameters. From the report of A.B. Smith and coworkers (1982)

Description of headache[a]	Association found with[b]	Trend found[c]
Occurring during tension, worry and/or stress	Years of VDT work	Negative
Associated with work	Bothersome visual aspects of VDT	Positive
	Workplace light	Positive
	Job hard, fast	Positive
With eye strain symptoms	Bothersome visual aspects (probably workstation)	Positive
Superficially located	Eye shift mode	Positive
With double or blurry vision	Hours of VDT work	Negative

[a] Only headache categories for which a significant association was found are given here. For 12 categories, no association was found, e.g. "headaches not associated with work", "headache made worse primarily by coughing or sneezing", "headaches that radiate into shoulders, accompanied by muscle tenseness", etc.

[b] Only factors for which a significant association with a headache category was found.

[c] Negative = significant negative association found. Positive = significant positive association found.

Relations between headache and some aspects of VDT work. The occurrence of reported headaches was higher for data-entry than for conversational-mode operators, according to Elias and colleagues (1982). An increase in headache occurrence with working time at VDTs was found by Wallin and coworkers (1983). However, A.B. Smith and coworkers (1982), reported that the number of hours/week at VDTs was negatively correlated with headaches preceeded or accompanied by blurry or double vision. Knave and coworkers (1985a), found that headaches were associated on one specific day with total working time, but not with the time spent looking at the screen. On another day, however, with a longer working time (in general), headaches were not associated with total working time.

A.B. Smith and coworkers (1982) found a positive correlation between bothersome visual aspects of VDT work and some headache types as already indicated in Table 3. Headaches were strongly associated with eye discomfort according to Knave and coworkers (1985a), and also in their investigation women reported more headaches than men.

5.3.4 Stress related disorders

A number of stress factors are apparent in VDT work, related to the work environment, the job content and organizational conditions, and also influenced by the worker's capacity, need and expectations, as well as customs, culture and extra-job conditions. A discussion on these factors as they have been noted in VDT work is found on pp. 70-85. A general discussion on these factors can be found, for example, in the ILO/WHO report (1984) and Dy (1985).

The consequences of these psychosocial factors as they appear in VDT work in terms of physiological, psychological and behavioural events, as well as the possibility of persistent health consequences will be discussed here. In the present publication, these consequences are referred to collectively as "stress-related disorders".

Psychological disturbances noted in the VDT literature are anger, frustation, nervousness, irritability, anxiety, confusion and depression. Behavioural changes, such as the effects on sleep pattern and appetite have been studied in a few reports. Some physiological consequences have also been considered in the context of psychosocial factors, such as gastrointestinal disturbances, muscular tension, changes in cardiovascular functions, sweating and excretion of catecholamines. The introduction of VDTs may have different physiological consequences at different times. An example is a stimulating period during introduction and training, which may change into monotony and qualitative underload during later routine operations (Johansson, 1986).

5.3.4.1 Psychological disturbances

A problem in evaluating the reports in this area is the lack of standards of assessment of the disorders; especially since data often originate from questionnaire response. While some studies use standardized profiles such as POMS (profile of mood states), other studies report only the questionnaire answers.

Occurrence among VDT operators. High occurrences of psychological disturbances are found among VDT operators, as they are in many other jobs, see the ILO/WHO report (1984). In the study by Elias and coworkers (1982), the occurrence of disturbances such as anxiety, irritability and depression varied between 25% and 70% for VDT operators. In the study made by Ghinghirelli (1982), anxiety and depressive disorders were reported by approximately 40%, while Johansson and Aronsson (1984) reported that irritation was found among 14% in the VDT operators.

Inadequate sleep patterns have been reported by Elias and coworkers (1982) for 15% to 45% of the VDT operators.

Differences between VDT operators and controls. A number of studies have been made on the possible differences between VDT operators and controls as to the occurrences of psychological and behavioural events. The results have been varied, presumably due in part to the wide variety of job situations, which are not distinctly separated by the descriptors 'VDT' versus 'non-VDT' jobs.

According to some studies (Canadian Labour Congress, 1982; Frank, 1983), irritation was associated with the use of VDT. In the study by Lewis and coworkers (1982) fatigue was not reported more frequently among VDT operators

than among controls, while nervousness (34% versus 21%) was more frequent.
Irritability was also found more frequently among VDT operators, but the
difference (45% versus 35%) was not stastistically significant. In other
studies (Dainoff et al., 1981; Johansson & Aronsson, 1984), the influence of
unreliable equipment or prolonged response times on irritation was reported,
according to the authors, presumably linked to lack of user control. See also
a discussion on this by MacKay and Cox (1984).

In contrast to these findings, two studies found no positive association
between psychological disturbances and VDT work. Binaschi and coworkers
(1982), found that fatigue (including nervousness and anxiety) was not
significantly higher among VDT-operators than among controls. A negative
correlation was seen between VDT work per se and mood disturbances, in the
study by Sauter and colleagues (1983a), where the effects of other factors
such as job demands had been separated from the effects of the VDT.

In some other studies, symptoms were found more frequently among certain
groups of VDT operators only (compared to corresponding controls) (Canadian
Labour Congress, 1982; Johansson & Aronsson, 1984; Murray et al., 1981b) . In
one study by Heron (1982), VDT clerical workers had higher 'stress points'
than controls, with VDT-using programmers having the lowest 'stress points',
while in the study by the Canadian Labour Congress, (1982), telephone
operators and reservation agents using VDTs showed more irritability than
corresponding non-VDT workers, but clerical workers did not report differences
related to use of VDTs or not. (Note that job classifications may vary.)

5.3.4.2 Behavioural consequences of work on visual display terminals

Sleeplessness and loss of appetite were found more frequently among VDT
operators than controls, according to the Canadian Labour Congress study
(1982). Engel (1982), and Lewis and coworkers (1982) also found that sleep
disturbances were correlated with VDT use.

Knave and colleagues (1985a), did not find any differences between VDT and
non-VDT users in alcohol consumption or cigarette smoking.

5.3.4.3 <u>Physiological consequences of psychosocial factors</u>

Occurrences of psychosomatic symptoms as reported by Elias and coworkers (1982) varied between 15% and 50% of the VDT operators. Symptoms reported were palpitations, constipation, chest pain, and other lower gastrointestinal disturbances, which the authors classified as flatulence.

<u>Differences between VDT operators and controls</u>. In the Canadian Labour Congress study (1982), tiredness (78% versus 68%) and dizziness (33% versus 24%) were more commonly found among VDT operators than controls. Occurrences were 'at least once in the last three months'. When daily occurrences were specified, the same cluster existed, but with lower rates. The authors point out, that although a significantly higher proportion of VDT users experience these problems, the occurrences among non-VDT workers were also high. These differences were found for professional, data-entry and 'dialogue' groups, but not for clerical groups. The data were the results of a questionnaire study, without analysis being performed on the impact of confounding or other contributing factors. When multifactorial methods were used to analyse this impact on telephone operators within this cohort, psychosomatic symptoms were not found to correlate with VDT use, according to Rowland (1984).

Neither dizziness nor irregular menstrual periods were found by Lewis and colleagues (1982) to be more frequent among VDT operators than controls. Sauter and coworkers (1983a) found no significant correlation between VDT work <u>per se</u> and ill health symptoms, after adjustments for the effects of other factors.

Gastrointestinal disturbances were more common among some VDT groups with intermediate VDT work duration, compared to controls and to VDT operators working more than 50% at VDTs according to Johansson and Aronsson (1984).

In the study by Johansson and Aronsson (1984), several physiological measures of stress reactions were measured for 21 individuals, both VDT operators and controls; heart rate, blood pressure and excretion of adrenaline and noradrenaline in the urine. All individual levels were reported as a percentage of levels on days off work. The average work-day adrenaline levels were higher among VDT operators than among controls, and the differences

remained also in the evenings after work. Increases in blood pressures among
VDT operators were found, but must be interpreted with caution, due to
methodological problems in that only one off-work measurement could be made.
No significant differences in noradrenaline levels or heart rates were found.

The adrenaline levels were, before noon, higher among VDT operators than
in controls, while the opposite was true in the afternoons (see Fig. 8).
These variations correlated with self-reported changes in anxiety, fatigue and
stress. The VDT operators reported that they worked hard in the mornings - in
case the system broke down, which often lead to lighter workloads in the
afternoons, while non-VDT workers reported increased workloads during the
afternoon - letters left to type late in the day, etc. (Johansson & Aronsson,
1984).

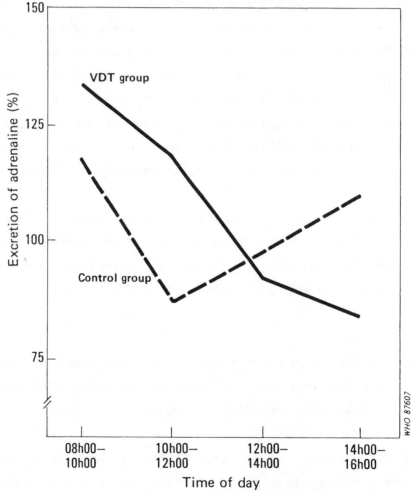

Fig. 8: Urinary mean excretion of adrenaline during the workday for the VDT
operators and for a control group. Values given are a percentage of those
measured at home during a non-working day. From Johansson and Aronsson (1984).

5.3.4.4 The possibility of persistent health consequences

A recent study by the North Carolina Occupational Safety & Health Project,
(1985) has suggested that angina (reported as chest pain in the questionnaire)
may be more common among VDT-operators than controls, but that this difference
was only noticed in jobs where workers stated that they had high control over
their work (16% versus 4%). For those who did not report "control" over their
work, the frequency of chest pain was independent of VDT work (approximately
15%). The fact that these results are the response to self-reporting
questionnaires and that the response rate was 40% should be pointed out;
comparisons of the rates of chest pain found in this study (4% to 16%) with
the rates of angina found in the general population is therefore difficult (as
yet the data have only been reported in a summary).

5.3.4.5 Relations between stress disorders and potential stress factors found
         during work on visual display terminals

Job content and organisational conditions. As can be inferred from
Section 5.3.4.3 above, job types and job stress factors are probably of major
importance in determining stress disorders. Johansson (1986) examined four
descriptors of heavy mental load in these respects; quantitative overload (too
much work) and qualitative underload (too simple and unqualified work) in
combination with inadequate operator control and social support. These four
descriptors are often found among operators doing repetitive data-entry work,
which as a group often experience an excessive mental load. For example,
Schleifer (1986) found a significant build-up of mood disturbances among
operators performing data-entry work.

Sauter (1984) found that uncertainty about employment was positively
correlated with mood disturbances, illness symptoms and job dissatisfaction.
Neither job control nor social support were associated with mood or illness
symptoms, but they were negatively associated with job dissatisfaction. Work
load demands were positively associated with illness symptoms, but not with
job satisfaction or mood symptoms.

Telephone operators placing international calls were somewhat more
susceptible to strain, ostensibly due to cross-cultural differences while

placing calls (Wilkins, 1983). Less control over work, higher job pressure, lower job satisfaction, higher degree of monitoring or incorrect spacing of workers were associated with higher stress (Canadian Labour Congress, 1982). These investigators did not, however, perform any analysis as to potential confounding factors.

Schleifer (1986) found that slow system response times caused increased levels of frustration, impatience and irritation. Wage incentive systems did not, by themselves, cause changes in mood disturbances. However, in combination with fast response times, wage incentives resulted in an increased level of rush compared to nonincentives. In combination with slow response time, wage incentives resulted in increased frustration and impatience. Thus, wage incentives did produce an increased sense of time urgency.

Duration of VDT work. No association (by multifactorial analysis) was found between hours of daily VDT use and mood or illness symptoms (Sauter, 1984). In the study by Johansson and Aronsson (1984), operators with intermediate VDT job-duration reported a greater incidence of gastrointestinal symptoms, compared to those with a shorter or a longer VDT job-duration (as already mentioned earlier).

In another study by Dainoff and coworkers (1981), the VDT-operators were generally fairly positive towards their jobs, but did report more tension and fatigue towards the end of the working day.

In an investigation by Marek and Noworol (1986), various indicators were used to assess mental arousal and fatigue during different types of data-entry work. Indicators used were: pupil diameter, blinking and search stimulation movements. In addition, fatigue was examined. The 35 subjects were young, and performed either monotonous or varying tasks, with a 15 min rest break after every 50 min of work. Operators doing varying tasks had increased arousal during the first part of the day, followed by a decrease in the afternoon (as indicated by pupil diameter), while monotonous task operators experienced a low level of arousal and a decrease throughout the day (apart from a small temporary increase after about 2.5 h of work). Fatigue increased throughout the day for both types of data-entry jobs.

In another study on data-entry workers, Floru and Cail (1986) examined the effects of work being (1) continuous at self-pace, (2) the same but under time pressure, and (3) with rest breaks included. Various psychophysiological effects were monitored (performance, EEG, heart rate, etc.). Arousal and performance declined with time during continuous work, but efforts of self-arousal (cerebral compensation) were also suggested. Rest breaks appeared to restore arousal, without the need for such compensation efforts. The authors suggested that similar effects could probably be achieved by varying the work content. Wennberg and Voss (1986) investigated subjects performing intensive work with videocoding. EEG recordings showed a relationship between vigilance and performance, but there were few effects of job conditions (breaks, morning compared to afternoon) on vigilance, which may have been due to large individual variations.

Interruptions in work routine. Wallin and coworkers (1983) reported that 81% of questioned VDT-operators experienced "disturbances" due to long and varying waiting times. Of 95 respondents, 63% would have liked to maximize waiting time to 5 seconds, while only 5% could accept waiting times of more than 30 seconds according to Johansson and Aronsson, (1984). The report of Schleifer (1986) also deals with the combination of response time and wage incentive systems.

Some studies of the consequences of unscheduled breaks in system operations have been reported. Considerable concern ("vehemence") was expressed at one study location towards the frequency with which their system would break down, resulting in failures to complete jobs, especially during telephone inquiries (Dainoff et al., 1981).

In the study by Johansson and Aronsson (1984), 60% of 95 VDT-operators, working more than 50% of their working time at VDTs, could not relax during unscheduled breaks, compared to about 10% of those working only occasionally at VDTs. During one unscheduled break (duration 3.5 h), the urinary levels of adrenaline and also the diastolic blood pressure were significantly higher than during normal VDT work. Irritation, stress and tiredness were also increased during this break period. The study was performed once on six individuals (Johansson & Aronsson, 1984).

Physical parameters of VDT work. Among professional VDT operators there
was a positive correlation between the level of complaints of several physical
VDT parameters and the level of complaints about mood disturbances, according
to Stammerjohn and coworkers (1981). The physical parameters related to
emotion and mood complaints were screen brightness, angle, height, glare and
flicker as well as noise from the VDT. The interrelationship with eye
discomforts was not evaluated. In theory, a chain relationship between glare,
eye discomfort, and mood disturbances is possible. Such relationships are
supported by the findings of Sauter and coworkers (1983b). However, the fact
that noise complaints were related to mood, as noted above by Stammerjohn and
colleagues, does suggest that more direct relationships may also exist.

Opinions have been expressed by Wallach (1982) concerning possible health
implications of changes in air ion concentrations, especially concerning
psychological disturbances. Apparently, there is no research which has
systematically examined such associations in VDT-situations. However, levels
of air ions were examined by Knave and coworkers (1985b), in 400 VDT
workstations in a number of locations, and were found to vary between about
10^8 and 5.10^8 ions/m^3. These levels are much lower than those for which
the possiblity of effects might be considered (more than 10^{10} ions/m^3)
according to Backman (1979) (see also Section 5.2.4.2 for further
discussion). Furthermore, Knave and coworkers (1985b) did not find any
consistent relation between air ion levels and physical discomforts.

5.3.5 Skin disorders

Attention has been given the possibility that work with VDTs may involve
a risk of developing facial skin problems. So far, a number of case reports
have appeared, describing facial disorders among VDT operators, primarily
in Norway, Sweden and the United Kingdom. In addition, the results of
a few epidemiological studies have also included information on skin
disorders.

5.3.5.1 Occurrence of skin disorders

Case reports of observed facial disorders. The Norwegian rash episodes
usually started after a few hours of exposure, and began with itching,
followed by erythema and sometimes also papules. These phenomena were usually
confined to the cheeks, and were usually graded as weak (Lindén & Rolfsen,
1981; Nilsen, 1982; Tjönn, 1984). Minor desquamations were frequent (Tjönn,
1984). These cases could not be characterized as either allergic contact
dermatitis, photosensitive dermatitis, or rosacea (Nilsen, 1982). No atopic
dermatitis in childhood, or among relatives was found in these cases (Tjönn,
1984).

The British cases also showed erythema and papules, but the investigators
found some resemblance to rosacea (Rycroft & Calnan, 1984).

Some reported Swedish cases were first diagnosed as having rosacea or
Civatte's poikiloderma (Lidén & Wahlberg, 1985a). A further 100 cases (95
women, 5 men) referred because of a suspected VDT relationship, have been
reported (Lidén & Wahlberg, 1986). Diagnoses included acne (14 subjects),
rosacea or perioral dermatitis (14), seborrhoeic dermatitis (22), atopic
dermatitis (8), telangiectases (10), and normal skin (6). The authors
emphasized, that although frequencies of occurrences among VDT-operators could
not be determined from case reports, the diversity of diagnoses among these
cases agreed with that of the general population.

Stenberg (1986) reported on nine cases of skin troubles among 14 VDT
operators in an office adjacent to a paper pulp mill in northern Sweden. Five
had rashes resembling rosacea, three facial erythema and one had only sensory
symptoms. All suffered from itching, burning and swelling of the skin. The
appearance coincided with VDT work. Two of 12 workers not engaged on VDTs
reported slight but similar symptoms.

One case has been diagnosed by another physician as having solar
elastosis, as evidenced by microscopic examination, which is described as
commonly being caused by UV radiation (Lagerholm, 1985). A diagnosis of
Civette's poikiloderma was also made by this physician; this case was accepted

by a local Swedish Worker Compensation Board as being a work-related disease.[1] In an earlier investigation by Kligman (1969), microscopically determined elastosis solaris was, however, found to be very common - the study reported 100% occurrence among those 40-49 years old, that the author attributed primarily to exposure to sunshine.

Epidemiological studies on skin rashes. An epidemiological study of the occurrence of skin disorders by Frank (1983) failed to find any differences between VDT-users and nonusers in newspaper offices in Canada and USA. Another study by Murray and coworkers (1981b) found in one of three locations investigated an increase in skin rashes, itching skin or allergic skin reactions in VDT operators compared with controls. Two surveys have included questions on skin rashes; responses from VDT-operators were 5.8% as reported by Evans (1985) and 7.9% as reported by the US National Association of Working Women (1984).

Knave and coworkers (1985a), found skin disorders to be more frequently reported by VDT operators (36%) than by controls (25%). Of individuals reporting recent skin disorders from this study, 96 were called in for a medical examination (Lidén & Wahlberg, 1985a). Of these, 74 were finally available for diagnosis, and 15 different diagnoses were made (objectively or anamnestically), which were arranged in four groups. One group (seborrhoeic dermatitis, acne, rosacea and perioral dermatitis) was found more frequently among VDT-operators than controls. None of the diagnosed cases was similar to the Norwegian cases described earlier.

In another study by Lidén & Wahlberg (1985b), a questionnaire was sent to 179 rosacea or perioral dermatitis patients (no controls were involved). Of these 42 worked with VDTs, and a possible relationship between aggravation of rosacea and VDT work was suggested (see further below).

---

[1] In the Swedish insurance legislation, it is not necessary to demonstrate a causal relationship between occupational exposure and a disease in order to accept the disease as work-related. It is sufficient that the evidence against such a relationship is not stronger than that in favour of it.

All these studies discussed above had methodological difficulties. These include low response rates (Frank, 1983; Murray et al., 1981a, b), or the use of self-selected populations (surveys by Evans [1985] and the US National Association of Working Women [1984]). In these surveys, as in the study by Lidén and Wahlberg (1985b), control groups were not used. In the study by Lidén and Wahlberg (1985a), which was performed on part of the cohort defined in the study by Knave and coworkers (1985a), no dermatological examination was performed on subjects who did not report skin disorders, thus the study did not identify possible false negatives.

Because of these difficulties, the question of whether VDT work causes skin disorders, cannot be fully evaluated from these studies.

5.3.5.2 Possible causes of the skin disorders

Relation of these disorders to VDT work duration. Workers with skin disorders consistently claimed to have developed a rash only when working with VDTs and that the rash disappeared away from VDT work (Lidén & Rolfsen, 1981; Nilsen, 1982; Rycroft & Calnan, 1984; Tjönn, 1984). Provocation tests of some patients have been carried out, with varying results. Five patients were placed in front of a VDT for three work periods, without any rash developing (Nilsen, 1982). Another investigator, however, reported successful provocation of facial disorders in two operators (Lidén & Rolfsen, 1981).

In the epidemiological study by Knave and coworkers (1985a), no significant relationship was found between rash occurrence and working time, and no such relation found when specific diagnoses were considered (Lidén & Wahlberg, 1985a).

In a rosacea questionnaire study by Lidén & Wahlberg (1985b), eight patients (of 42 working with VDTs) suggested that their rosacea became worse during VDT work.

Other factors that may be involved. One consistent observation in many case reports has been the coincidence of the facial disorders with dry weather (low relative humidity) and with the frequent occurrence of electrostatic phenomena (Lidén & Rolfsen, 1981; Nilsen, 1982; Rycroft & Calnan, 1984; Tjönn, 1984).

Some investigations of ionizing and nonionizing (UV) radiation levels were made on the VDTs at which some of the cases had been working, and the levels were found to be very low to nondetectable (Nilsen, 1982; Rycroft & Calnan, 1984). In the epidemiological study by Knave and coworkers (1985b), no correlation between ambient UV levels and the frequency of skin disorders could be found.

Electrostatic fields and skin disorders. The localization of skin disorders to only a few offices, their occurrence in only certain individuals and the noted correlation with low humidity, have lead to the suggestion that these skin disorders (as reported in case reports) could be explained by enhanced ambient aerosol exposure due to electrostatic fields (Cato Olsen, 1981).

An investigation was performed by Cato Olsen (1981) in Bergen, Norway, where the six rash cases referred to by Nilsen (1982) worked. High electrostatic fields were found around some of the "rash-prone" VDTs, but also among other VDTs, where no rash episodes had been reported. These high electrostatic body potentials were in offices were rash episodes had occurred, but were found equally on rash-prone operators, non-rash-prone operators, and also on the investigators. In an experimental part of the study, the deposition of excess aerosol material, compared to controls, increased with increasing electrostatic fields between the VDT and the operator (Cato Olsen, 1981). The author suggested that electrostatic fields, especially influenced by the electrostatic charge on the operator (possibly augmented by the electrostatic charge of the VDT), enhanced particle deposition on the face, and that, depending on the nature of the aerosol contaminants, skin reactions to these contaminants might occur in susceptible individuals. In further investigations (Cato Olsen, 1986), measurements in model situations similar to those with occurring static electricity problems (i.e. with fairly high operator charges) disclosed that the electrostatic field from the VDT made only a minor contribution to the field in the vicinity of the face.

According to this suggestion, the air humidity would be important, since the electrostatic charge on the operator is strongly dependent on air humidity. Neither in Knave and colleagues study (1985b) nor in that of Murray and coworkers (1981b) were any obvious relationships found between air humidity and the occurrences of skin disorders. These authors, however, pointed out that the measured humidity may not be representative of either seasonal or year-round conditions.

In the epidemiological study by Knave and colleagues (1985b), neither the electrostatic field nor the body potential from the VDTs was correlated with subjectively reported skin disorders. When specific diagnoses were considered (Lidén & Wahlberg, 1985a), these again failed to show any relationship with the electrostatic field from the VDT, but in the one group which appeared to be possibly VDT-related (seborrhoeic or perioral dermatitis, acne and rosacea), significantly more positive body potentials were noted compared with other groups.

In this context, an experimental study has been performed by the Swedish National Institute of Radiation Protection (Bengtsson, 1986) to investigate the increase in radon daughter exposure of an operator with a body potential sitting in front of a VDT with an electrostatic field. The results indicated that under the experimental conditions used, the exposure would be increased by a factor of 1.6, based on year-average. The author did not consider this enhanced radon daughter exposure to be sufficient to cause skin damage. In a cluster reported by Stenberg (1986), the presence of indoor air particles and volatile substances are currently being examined. Further experiments are underway by several investigators to elucidate the possible influence of various air contaminants on these skin disorders.

Attempts made to prevent facial rashes among rash-prone operators. From the observations given above and from theoretical consideration (see Knave et al., 1985b), it appears that measures to limit the body potentials may possibly be of some interest when attempting to prevent some skin disorders. Decreasing or eliminating the electrostatic field from the VDT is, on the other hand, not expected to interfere with development of skin disorders depending on aerosol deposition.

Some intervention results are of interest. Increasing the air humidity (to about 50%) has reduced rash reactions markedly. Elimination of static electricity-prone carpets in combination with high humidity resulted in the disappearance of the facial disorders (Lindén & Rolfsen, 1981). These findings are in agreement with the aerosol deposition hypothesis. However, the placement of a grounded metal or wire mesh screen, or a water screen (a glass container filled with an electrolyte solution), between the VDT and the operator has in some cases reduced the skin disorders (Lindén & Rolfsen, 1981). Other attempts to reduce skin disorders by eliminating the electrostatic field from the VDT have not been successful (Stenberg, 1986; Bergqvist et al., 1986).

It should be pointed out, that the diversity of the types of skin problems found among VDT-operators indicates that a single factor or factor combination is not likely to explain all these skin problems. While the aerosol deposition hypothesis is a working hypothesis for some skin disorders, other findings, such as increased manifestation of rosacea or some other labile skin disorders, may possibly be explained by stress reactions.

5.3.6 Photosensitive epilepsy

Another physiological effect will be briefly discussed; the possibility of inducing photosensitive epileptic seizures. The literature on this phenomenon in connection with VDTs is rather limited.

Cases of grand mal seizures have been observed in connection with television viewing. The phenomenon appears to be rare, however, and only a small fraction of the population (approximately 1/5000) appear to be at risk (Binnie et al., 1985; Jeavons et al., 1985; Wilkins, 1983). A few isolated cases of seizures while working at VDTs have been reported, but the investigators, Jeavons and coworkers (1985), noted that in one case, the person had a history of spontaneous seizures, and then had continued working with VDTs for two years without further seizures. The other case reported by the same authors could not be confirmed, since no evidence of photosensitivity was found.

It was suggested by Jeavons and coworkers (1985) and Binnie and colleagues (1985), that many VDT screens may be less likely to produce seizures than television screens, because of the absence of interlace, a lower flicker tendency, no apparent raster pattern, smaller screens and lower luminance. It was also noted, however, that changes in these parameters, as in graphic displays or use of domestic television sets as computer displays, etc., may

change this evaluation. One case of seizures in a boy using a domestic
television set to play computer games has been reported by Jeavons and
coworkers (1985). In a test series performed by Binnie and colleagues (1985),
a visual display unit with a short persistence phosphor consistently failed to
cause epileptiform activity in photosensitive subjects, while similar tests
using black-and-white television have caused epileptiform discharges in many
photosensitive subjects.

5.3.7 Adverse reproductive outcomes

The occurrence of several clusters of unusually high miscarriage or birth
defect rates among pregnant VDT operators has been reported. Discussion of
the possible influence of VDT work on pregnancy outcome has led to apprehension
and worry among VDT operators, and the need to investigate this possibility.

The basis for the concern about possible interactions between pregnancy
and VDT work will be examined in some detail, first in terms of the clusters
of adverse pregnancy outcomes that have appeared, secondly as regards the
possible factors in VDT work that could conceivably cause a teratogenic
effect, and finally as regards the results of epidemiological studies.

In the reported clusters, the outcomes under discussion were generally
confined to spontaneous abortion and congenital defects. Thus, studies have
by and large been centred on these outcomes. A brief discussion on
appropriate definitions is in order.

Spontaneous abortion. Spontaneous abortion is normally defined as the
involuntary termination of pregnancy prior to the end of the 28th week.
Spontaneous abortion occurring before the pregnancy has been recognized will
be manifested as infertility. Data from VDT operators are limited to
spontaneous abortion in recognized pregnancies. No study has been performed
on the fertility of VDT-workers.

The definitions and methods used to detect spontaneous abortion are
important, and ambiguity in this respect within a study is an important cause
of bias. The specific definitions used in this publication are those found in
the individual studies, e.g., use of self-reported spontaneous abortion as in

most studies, or registers of hospitalized spontaneous abortion as in the studies by Ericson and coworkers (1985a) and Källén (1985a).

The "normal" rate of spontaneous abortion in recognized pregnancies varies with not only the definition used, but also the number of confounding factors (age, etc., see pp. 147-148 below). The normal rate is usually reckoned to be 8-20% (Axelsson, 1983; Kajiwara, 1984; McDonald et al., 1983; McDonald, 1984).

Congenital defects. In this publication, the term congenital defects, is limited to significant or serious effects, generally implying defects that "seriously interfere with viability or physical well-being" (McDonald, 1984). The period of observation (detection) is also a limiting factor, in some studies thereby excluding defects with late manifestations.

As above, specific criteria within a study are important, and ambiguity will lead to problems of interpretation. In general, the rate of significant congenital defects is of the order of 1-4% (Elinson et al., 1980; McDonald, 1984; Saxén, 1981).

Other outcomes. Other outcomes that have been studied in some investigations are low birth weight and perinatal death. These are referred to when discussing individual studies. In the Swedish Register study (Källén, 1985a), the term birth defect implies one or several of: significant congenital defect, perinatal death and very low birth weight.

5.3.7.1 Reported clusters of spontaneous abortions or congenital defects

A number of "clusters" or high frequencies of spontaneous abortion or birth defects among groups of VDT operators have been reported mainly from Canada and the USA. Those found in the literature, and which occurred (at least in part) during 1979 and 1980 are shown in Table 4. Additional clusters have since appeared, a comment in 'Microwave News' in May 1984 (ANON: 1984) cited 11 clusters being "made public" (Millar, 1984; ANON: VDT News, 1984). Further cluster appearances have been reported by the US National Association of Working Women (1983). Clusters have also been reported from other countries, e.g., Australia, Denmark, Sweden, and the United Kingdom.

Table 4. Increased incidence of spontaneous abortion or congenital defects among groups of VDT-operators in Canada and the USA.   Only clusters that occurred (at least partly) in the period 1979-1980 are included[a].

Occurrence/place	Date	Events noted[b]
Sears Roebuck, Dallas, Texas	May 1979– June 1980	SA= 7/12 (ND= 1/12)
Defence Logistic Agency, Atlanta, Georgia	Oct. 1979– Oct. 1980	SA= 7/15 CD= 3/15
Toronto Star Toronto	May 1979– May 1980	CD= 4/7
Canadian Air Line, Dorval, Quebec	Feb. 1979– Feb. 1980	SA= 7/13
Old City Hall, Toronto	1980–1981	SA= 10/19
Surrey Memorial Hospital, British Columbia	May 1978– Oct. 1982	SA= 3/7 CD= 2/7 (PB= 1/7) (RD= 1/7)
Office of Solicitor-General, Ottawa	1979–1982	SA= 4/7 (PB= 1/7) (RD= 2/7)

[a] Additional clusters in Canada and the USA have since appeared in, e.g., Renton, Washington (3 adverse of 5), Alma, Michigan (17 adverse of 32), Atlanta, Georgia (6 adverse of 15), Great Neck, New York (6 adverse, total number of pregnancies in the period not stated), San Francisco, California (19 adverse of 48) and Gander, Newfoundland (3 adverse of 31). The rate of cluster appearances does not seem to have increased since 1979-1980. References to those tabulated and the later additional clusters may be found in Binkin et al., 1981; DeMatteo, 1984; Johnson & Melius, 1986; Labour Canada 1982; Landrigan et al., 1983; National Association of Working Women, 1983; Purdham, 1984; Sharma, 1984; ANON: VDT News, I & II, 1984; ANON: Microwave News, 1984.

[b] Number of occurrences/number of pregnant women working with VDTs in a (specified) group. Abnormally high incidences only noted. SA = spontaneous abortion, CD = congenital defect, ND = neonatal death, PB = premature birth, RD = respiratory disease.

Several clusters have been investigated by NIOSH (ANON: VDT News, I & II, 1984; ANON: VDT Microwave News, 1984) and (Johnson & Melius, 1986), the US Army Environmental Hygiene Agency [reported by Purdham (1984)] in the USA, by the City of Toronto (Elinson et al., 1980) and by the REMS (Sharma, 1984) in Canada, as well as by the National Board of Occupational Safety and Health in Sweden. Sharma (1984) reported that the the extremely-low-frequency electric and magnetic fields were recorded in one cluster location, that of the Surrey Memorial Hospital, Vancouver. The measuring technique, and these results, have, however, been criticized by Guy (1984) who also performed measurements around one of the units involved, and found the levels to be much lower. A critical review on this and also on the statistical bias was made by Mohanna and coworkers (1986).

In none of the other investigated clusters, could any specific factor be linked to the observed pregnancy outcomes. For the Toronto Star cluster, measurements were made for ionizing radiation, but none detected. Levels of non-ionizing radiation were very low or non-existent, well below existing standards (Elinson et al., 1980). The same results were found for the VDTs used at the Old City Hall, Toronto, where another cluster appeared. The makes tested by the US Bureau of Radiological Health, and found to emit low but measurable X-ray levels during extreme conditions (Section 5.2.2.2) were not used in Canada. For a review, see Purdham (1984).

In the Sears-Roebuck cluster investigation, a follow up study one year later revealed four new pregnancies, all of which resulted in term births (Landrigan et al., 1983). In the Toronto Star cluster (four congenital defects), there were four different defects: underdeveloped eye, club-foot, cleft palate and "hole in the heart". (One mother reported a family history of cleft palate.) It has been argued that the diversity of these defects is not in accordance with the possibility of one single external factor as a cause of all these effects (Elinson et al., 1980).

The Runcorn study: A study was initiated at Runcorn, England, after the appearance of a cluster at a data processing centre. Of the 803 questionnaires sent to women employed at the office complex during 1974 and 1982, 72% were returned (Lee & McNamee, 1984). A total of 55 women became pregnant during a spell of working with VDTs (at least 10 h/week, 3 months prior and 3 months after conception), while 114 other women also became pregnant but did not work with VDTs. Eight exposed and six control pregnancies ended in miscarriages; for 13 exposed and 12 control pregnancies, the outcome was a stillbirth or a fetal abnormality (including minor abnormalities). The rates of miscarriage were higher among the exposed than among the control subjects (14.5% compared with 5.5%), although, as the authors point out, the miscarriage rate among the exposed agree well with in the normal rates in other studies. No test of significance was performed, since the group under study was "in effect, self-selected", being based on a reported cluster. The authors therefore stress that "inference concerning VDU workers as a whole would not necessarily be valid".

The Polish study: Another study was performed in two offices in Poland, one at the Lot airline offices and the other at a building construction bureau. According to available information, the study was apparently performed after the appearance of a cluster. Data on miscarriages were obtained by interview of company doctors. In the Lot offices (135 pregnancies), miscarriage rates were 36% among VDT-operators, compared to 16% among non-VDT operators. In the building construction bureau (50 pregnancies), no miscarriages occurred among the VDT operators compared to 15% among non-VDT operators. The authors suggested that heavy mental load during VDT work in the Lot offices was a possible factor contributing to the higher miscarriage rate (Mikolajczyk et al., 1986).

A plausible explanation of these recorded clusters is the combination of chance (random accumulation of a number of spontaneous abortion cases in a few of the many groups of pregnant women working with VDTs), together with the selective identification of only these groups. This possibility is examined in Annex 3, and the results are described below. The possibility of other explanations for these clusters, namely that of a specific VDT-related factor being involved, is considered in Sections 5.3.7.3 and 5.3.7.4.

5.3.7.2 Statistical evaluation of reported clusters

Spontaneous abortion. The six reported groups with high rates of spontaneous abortion occurring (in part) within the period summer 1979 – summer 1980, can be summarized as follows: number of pregnant women in each group : 7 – 19 (mean 12.2); percentage of spontaneous abortion in each group: 43 – 58% (mean 52%). There was no trend in the percentage values as the group size increased.

A model based on these data and suggestions has been presented by Bergqvist (1984) and is reprinted in Annex 3. The result indicates that the expected number of groups with high (more than 50%) spontaneous abortion rates is in agreement with or in excess of the number of observed (reported) groups. Similar conclusions have been made by Landrigan and coworkers (1983), Purdham (1984) and others. Landrigan and coworkers (1983) stated, after a detailed investigation of the Sears-Roebuck cluster, that the "findings may have been due to chance, given that no specific etiology was identified and that, in a sufficiently large number of groups of women, the likelihood is extremely high that at least some groups will have a high rate of adverse pregnancy outcome by chance alone".

Congenital defects. A similar analysis to that for the spontaneous abortion cases was made by Bergqvist (1984), see Annex 3. The expected number of groups with congenital defect rates similar to those observed was of the same order of magnitude as the number of observed groups.

Thus, the appearance of the reported clusters is not, by itself, evidence for an association between adverse pregnancy outcomes and VDT work, since such clusters are bound to occur by chance alone.

5.3.7.3 VDT-related factors and adverse reproductive outcomes

Investigating the possibility that VDT-related factors may be related to adverse outcomes of pregnancies, attention has been focused mainly on electromagnetic radiation and fields, but other factors such as stress or other components of the work environment have also been considered.

The intensities of electromagnetic radiation and fields usually measured around VDTs are not considered harmful, when evaluated from either existing occupational standards or known biological effect mechanisms, or when compared with the background levels found in other nonoccupational environments, as has previously been discussed on pp. 41-44. Some results pertinent to low frequency magnetic fields will be discussed in this section.

The emission of polychlorinated biphenyls (PCBs) from VDTs have been suggested in one report. This suggestion has, however, been repudiated by other investigations. VDTs are not considered a source of PCB emission. (This is discussed on p. 65.) Other factors have been suggested, e.g. ultrasound emission and ionization of the air. These suggestions, however, have not been presented with any supporting evidence or indications.

Stress disorders and pregnancy outcome. Some recent literature reviews by Mackay (1984) and Björseth and coworkers (1985) have suggested a link between stress disorders and spontaneous abortion. The latter group of authors suggested that worry about pregnancy outcome may itself be a possible stress factor. The possibility of a relationship between stress disorders and spontaneous abortion requires further attention, although the data available at present must be considered insufficient to suggest such a link.

The fact that stress factors may lead to altered behaviour (especially as regards smoking, alcohol use and other use of drugs etc.) and that these behaviours may affect pregnancy outcome have also been discussed (Källén, 1985b; MacKay, 1984).

In the section on stress disorders, no definite correlation between the use of VDT per se and stress disorders could be found. It is, however, prudent to emphasize that pregnant women should not be subjected to excessive stress or other adverse factors in the work environment, in VDT-jobs or in other jobs.

5.3.7.4 The effects of extra-low-frequency magnetic fields on chick embryogenesis

In a series of experiments, Delgado and coworkers have suggested the possibility that low intensity, low frequency magnetic fields with square pulse waves may adversely affect developmental processes (Delgado, 1982; Delgado et al., 1982; Trillo et al., 1983; Ubeda et al., 1983). In these experiments, fertilized hen eggs were exposed to pulsed magnetic fields (duration about 0.5 ms) with frequencies of 10, 100 or 1000 Hz, and intensities of 0.12, 1.2 or 12 μT. After 48 h the exposure was terminated, and the embryos were examined as to gross morphology of the intact embryo and histology of sections of the embryo.

In the first report by Delgado and coworkers (1982), 36 of 42 exposed eggs (compared with 4 of 26 controls) did show gross morphological abnormalities especially in the cephalic nervous system. The effects were most notable at 1.2 μT (compared to other amplitudes) and at 100 Hz (compared to the other frequencies).

In a subsequent report (Ubeda et al., 1983) a larger number of exposures were described and there was also some variation in pulse form. The repetition frequencies were 100 Hz, and the pulse duration 0.5 ms in all experiments. A significant increase in morphological abnormalities among exposed compared with control eggs was found only for certain pulse types, and at amplitudes of 0.4 μT or 1.0 μT. Other pulse types at these or other amplitudes caused no significant differences between exposed and control eggs.

It has been suggested that the relevant parameter for biological effects of such magnetic fields would be the time derivative of the magnetic field strength B: dB/dt. Examining the original data from Ubeda and coworkers (1983), no relationship between dB/dt and the abnormality ratios was observed by Bergqvist (1984). Subsequently, it was reported that some published data in the report by Ubeda and coworkers (1983) on rise-time (and thus calculated dB/dt) were in error - the rise-time was characteristic not of the exposure but of the instrument used to measure the field (ANON: Transmission/distribution & Safety Report, 1985).

Other groups have attempted to repeat these results. In one study, where the pulses had a rise-time of 10 μs, no differences were noted between exposed and control eggs (Maffeo et al. 1984). In one recently published paper, a partial success in replication has been reported. Magnetic fields of 100 Hz and various pulse forms (sine pulsed, square) resulted in an increase in malformed embryos compared to controls. According to the authors, the results do not, however, indicate that dB/dt (or the induced current) was related to the observed effects (Juutilainen & Saali, 1986). In studies performed by Tribukait and coworkers (1986), no effects of "square pulses" were seen on pregnant mice.

It has been suggested that if the results of Delgado and coworkers are accurate there could be effects of magnetic fields from VDTs on embryogenesis. This supposition has been based on the significant results that were seen for

24 and 200 mT/s, compared to dB/dt at VDTs (30 cm distance) of about 10 mT/s (see a discussion on this by Guy (1984) and Bergqvist (1984) and data by Paulsson and coworkers (1984). The results of Juutilainen and Saali (1986), suggest, however, that parameters other than dB/dt are related to effects.

However, other parameters distinguish between the pulse used by Delgado and coworkers and those found with VDTs as regards frequency, amplitude and pulse shape. This is noteworthy, since the Delgado group reported the existence of frequency windows, i.e., the effects decreased at other tested frequencies - higher and lower than 100 Hz. Marriott and Stuchly (1985) reached the following conclusions: "Although one or two parameters of the exposure fields employed in these studies are similar to those around VDTs, there are significant differences in numerous other parameters. Any extrapolation of the results of these studies to exposure of VDT operators can only be considered tenuous". Guy (1984) made a similar conclusion: "This comparison is based on similarity of the magnitude and rise times of the pulses used by Delgado with those of VDT magnetic emissions. However, the evidence for such speculation is weakened by the following facts: (a) The frequency of the Delgado magnetic pulses is over 150 times lower than those emitted by VDTs; (b) the width of the Delgado pulses is 10 times greater than those emitted by VDTs; (c) Delgado obtained nonsignificant effects with pulses of the same rise time and amplitude as those that produced significant effects."

Effects of magnetic pulses of saw-tooth form on embryos. One study on the possibility of teratogenic effects of saw-tooth pulses, similar to those found around VDTs, is being performed at the Karolinska Institute in Sweden. Some preliminary results have appeared (Tribukait et al., 1986). Pregnant mice were exposed to saw-tooth pulses (frequency 20 kHz, amplitude $1 \mu T$ (group III) and $15 \mu T$ (group IV) and a fall-time of $5 \mu sec$. The exposure was 24 h/day during the first 15 days of the 21-day pregnancy. According to the data up to January 1986, in group IV, seven malformed fetuses (3%) were noted compared to 2 (0.6%) in the control group. The number of dead fetuses (dead after cessation of exposure) was 0 (0%) in the exposed group compared with 5 (1.5%) in the control group - all percentages related to the total number of implants. Different interpretations of these data have been put forward: first, separate consideration of the dead and malformed fetuses might indicate a possible increase in malformations and a possible decrease in fetal deaths (the first observations were noted by the authors); secondly, a combination of living malformed and dead fetuses does not indicate any effect, and thirdly, considering the large number of comparisons made, these preliminary results may have been caused by chance.

Since January 1986, additional experiments have been undertaken, and the results were presented in May 1986 at the International Scientific Conference on Work with Display Units, in Stockholm. In the total material, there were no longer any significant differences between group IV and the controls. In the added material, the percentages of malformed fetuses were identical in group IV and the control group (2.0-2.1%), and the percentage of deat fetuses were also identical (1.1-1.2%). Some differences remained in external malformation, the added material contained two umbilicial hernias (1.1%) in group IV compared to one (0.4%) in the control group.

The exposure levels used for group IV (15 μT - 3000 mT/s) were considerably higher that those of VDT-operators (less than 0.2 μT, less than 100 mT/s, 76 cm distance). Extrapolation of the animal data to human subjects is, however, very difficult, since the possible mechanisms (and responsible parameters - B or dB/dt or something else? are unknown.

This study is continuing, and further data are expected. A similar study is being planned by another group. The data presented so far from this study are not considered to indicate that pulsed magnetic fields are a risk factor during VDT work (NIOSH, 1986). This is based on the uncertainty as to interpretation (discussed above) and the levels used.

In another study on the effects of saw-tooth pulsed magnetic fields on chick embryogenesis (Sandström et al., 1986), using exposure conditions identical to those of Tribukait and coworkers (1986) described above, no differences between exposed and control eggs were seen.

In the study by Mikolajczyk and colleagues (1986), 10 male rats were situated in front of a television set. Following sacrifice of the experimental animals, the authors noted a lower testicle weight among exposed rats compared to 10 control rats. However, the relative differences were not significant, and were furthermore equal to differences in body weights (recorded before the experiment). Thus, there is no basis for a suggestion that exposure to a television set caused a decrease in testicular weights.

Conclusions. Present knowledge does not support the conclusion that physical or chemical factors may be risk factors for adverse pregnancy outcome in women engaged in work with VDTs. Some suggested factors do, however, require further research (Section 5.4).

5.3.7.5 Research studies on pregnancy outcomes

Another approach to the question of adverse pregnancy outcomes among VDT operators is to conduct an epidemiological study. A number of such retrospective studies have been performed and a list of completed studies is presented in Table 5.

When evaluating these studies, a number of problems inherent in studies of this kind must be considered. Primarily these problems are concerned with the possibility of bias influencing the results. Different sources of bias were briefly discussed by Knill-Jones (1984) and some of his points reviewed here (with some added comments).

(i) The outcome of one pregnancy will have an effect on the next; one miscarriage predisposes to a further miscarriage. This may be a bias, if a full obstetric history is not included.

(ii) Comparing currently working women with non-working women, the outcome of previous pregnancies will to some degree determine whether the woman will continue work or not. Thus, there is a tendency for working women to have higher miscarriage rates (selection having occurred). This is of importance in cohort/cross-sectional studies, where overestimates of spontaneous abortion rates thus may occur.

(iii) Failure to adjust for factors that are known to affect pregnancy outcome (e.g. maternal age, parity, smoking, etc.) may introduce bias. Thus, a careful analysis can not be based on crude percentage data.

(iv) Uncertain endpoints are a serious problem when studying miscarriages, since uncertainty may exist in distinguishing between an early miscarriage or a late menstruation. Studies have shown that unconfirmed miscarriages can be overreported in exposed groups. Differences in diagnostic criteria (of malformations for example) between different physicians and hospitals or between different registers (also with time) may also contribute to bias, unless checked for matching.

(v) Different response tendencies are influenced by the fact of exposure. In case-control studies, different estimates of exposure may occur - overemphasized for cases or underemphasized for control (different tendency to "forget"). In cohort studies, uncertainty of endpoints may produce a response bias (both types have been documented). A low overall response rate does thus diminish the possibility of drawing conclusions from the data.

(vi) Induced abortions include a measure of uncertainty into calculations of rate of spontaneous abortions.

The essential elements which were used by the WHO Working Group on Occupational Health Aspects in the Use of Visual Display Terminals for their evaluation were:

- response rate and size of the study;
- possibility of confounding factors being analysed; and
- administrative aspects of data sources, registers, questionnaires/ interviews, possibility of self-selection.

Table 5. Studies on pregnancy outcome among VDT operators

Study	Type of study[a]	Pregnancies Year	Number	Reference[b]
Canadian Labour Congress	Cohort, N	prior to 1982	108[k]	R: Canadian Labour Congress, 1982
US Newspaper Guild	Cohort[c]	1977–82[d]	[c],[k]	R: Frank, 1983
Montreal, Canada (first previous)[e]	Cohort, C	prior to 1982	14 708	C: McDonald et al., 1983
Montreal (past)[e]	Cohort, C	prior to 1982	3 863	C: McDonald et al., 1984
Montreal (current)[d]	Cohort, C	1981–82	3 799	C: McDonald et al., 1984
Osaka, Japan	Cohort, N	prior to 1984	50	R: Kajiwara, 1984
Swedish National Insurance	Cohort, N	1980–83[f]	4 347[f]	P: Ericson et al., 1985b
North Carolina, USA[g]	Cohort[h]	prior to 1985	[g]; [k]	R: North Carolina Safety and Health Project, 1985
South Australia	Case-control within cohort	1960–78	90	P: Lewis et al., 1982
Swedish Register	Case-control within cohort	1980–81	1 447	P: Källén, 1985a; 1985b
Finnish Register	Case-control	1976–83	2 950	P: Kurppa et al., 1984; 1985
9 to 5 Campaign	Poll[i]	prior to 1984	206	R: US National Association of Working Women, 1983
Health & Safety at Work	Poll[i]	prior to fall 1985	435[k]	R: Evans, 1985

<u>a</u> No differentiation is made here between cohort and cross-sectional study. For cohort/cross-sectional studies, comparison group is also indicated: C= compared to non-VDT workers within the cohort; N= compared to expected (national data) etc.

<u>b</u> P = published in scientific journal. R = report. C = conference proceedings.

<u>c</u> No comparison made due to insufficient data. Number of pregnancies, total and separated into VDT-workers or not, have not been given in the report, a rough estimate of the total is about 150 (see below).

<u>d</u> Earlier pregnancies, back to the 1940s, also reported.

<u>e</u> For descriptions of subcohorts within the Montreal study, see below.

<u>f</u> Spontaneous abortion from 1980-81 only. Some pregnancies also included in the Swedish Register study.

<u>g</u> Few details given in the report, the number of pregnancies, e.g. was not stated.

<u>h</u> The study compared individuals working more than 50% of their time at VDTs, with individuals working less than 50% at VDTs, or not working with VDTs at all.

<u>i</u> These studies collected self-administrated questionnaire response from VDT-workers only, see further discussion below.

<u>k</u> Including wives of men working at VDTs.

Canadian Labour Congress Study (1982). In this questionnaire study, the
VDT-respondents (1067 women) reported 61 pregnancies, 47 normal, 13
miscarriages and one birth defect. The data also included data on wives of
male respondents, and reported as 3.2% birth defects (expected 4-8%) and 14%
miscarriages (expected 15-20%), observed adverse pregnancy outcome rates were
thus similar to the expected rates. Regarding only the women respondents,
neither the miscarriage rate nor the malformation rate differed significantly
from the expected values.

The Newspaper Guild Study (Frank, 1983). In a study of 2800 newspaper
workers in North America, a number of questions were asked as to reproductive
outcomes. In total 1047 responses (40%) were obtained, 542 of which were from
women; 67% of them used VDTs. Unfortunately, the report does not give
information as to the number of pregnancies involved; a crude estimate
based on other studies and evaluations (Bergqvist, 1984; Binkin et al., 1981;
Lee & McNamee, 1984) would be about 150 pregnancies.

From the period 1977-1982, 15 miscarriages were reported, seven among VDT-
operators, three among non-VDT operators, while five were "unknown". Keeping
in mind that 67% of the women were VDT-operators, these data do not indicate
any excess frequency of miscarriage among VDT-operators. The small numbers
do, however, preclude drawing any definite conclusion, especially since no
subdivision by age, etc., was possible and the exact fraction of pregnant
women working with VDTs was not given.

There was no evidence of premature birth or infant mortality due to VDT
exposure in this study. Birth defects could not be thoroughly evaluated,
owing to low numbers (three among the VDT-workers).

The Montreal Study (McDonald et al., 1983; 1984). In this study, women
attending 11 Montreal hospitals for childbirth, or because of a spontaneous
abortion, during a two-year period were interviewed. Each of these pregnancies
is labelled a current pregnancy in the following discussion. The interviews
concerned present and past pregnancies, socioeconomic data, data on the job
situation during each pregnancy, etc. (Institut de recherche en santé et en
sécurité du travail du Québec, 1983). Results from this study have been
presented at some conferences (McDonald et al., 1983; 1984). Each presentation
has used different subcohorts, and will thus be presented separately here.

In the first presentation (McDonald et al., 1983), the results of 14 708 interviews of women concerning their previous first pregnancy were given.[1] Of these 18.1% pregnancies ended in spontaneous abortion. Among VDT workers, the rate was 21.5%. The authors of the study express doubt about the validity of the VDT data: "This shorter interval for first conceptions ending in an abortion (to the present pregnancy), in conjunction with the trend to a wider use of VDTs systematically biases the relation between the two events...". A review evaluation of the data concurred. "It appears that the increase in spontaneous abortion among VDT workers noted in the study is fully explainable by this error (selective bias)" (Bergqvist, 1984).[2]

Work with a VDT did not correlate with any significant increase in the total birth defect rate compared to that of the total cohort, neither was any increase in the rate of low birth weights noted.

In the second presentation (McDonald et al., 1984), a subset of 7662 pregnancies was presented, from occupations including substantial VDT use. The results were separated into past (3863) and current (3799) pregnancies.

The rate of spontaneous abortion in past pregnancies was 21.3% (non-VDT-users), 23.3% (VDT use less than 15 h/week) and 29.0% (VDT use more than 15 h/week). However, spontaneous abortion among past pregnancies in this

---

[1] Thus, these data do concern the women's first pregnancy, but not the current one. Women for which the current pregnancy is their first one are thus not included in this subcohort, but are found below included in another subcohort.

[2] Basically, the problem is due to the fact that for a womam, who, for example, had a first conception in January 1982, and a second conception in May 1982, the first pregnancy must necessarily have ended in an abortion. Thus, the problem exists when conception of the first previous pregnancy and of the present pregnancy are close in time. Since VDT-occupation is increasing rapidly with time, pregnancies in VDT-workers will to a larger degree than others be exposed to this bias, which will result in an apparent increase in the reported rate of spontaneous abortions among VDT operators.

presentation suffered the same bias problem as mentioned above: of those
conceived before 1976, 10% ended in spontaneous abortion, while the percentage
was 68.9% for those conceived in 1981 and 100% of those conceived in 1982.
Detailed analysis of the data does not show any consistent difference between
VDT and non-VDT users as to abortion rates for each year (1974-1981).

Past pregnancies recorded 5.5% congenital defects among non-VDT-users,
while rates os 4.0 and 7.4% (respectively) were found among those with less
than 15 h/week and more to 15 h/week VDT work.

Data from current pregnancies do show some increase in spontaneous
abortion with VDT use: 5.7% (non-VDT), 8.2% (VDT less than 15 h/week) and 9.3%
(more than 15 h/weeks). The authors plan further analysis to evaluate this
finding, but do point out the possibility of response or selection bias (as
discussed above). Furthermore, in the study, "women working in sectors with
little use of VDTs had similar rates of abortion to those in sectors with
greater use of VDTs".

Congenital defects among current pregnancy did not show any significant
difference between VDT and non-VDT-workers.

In the final analysis of the data in the study relating to VDT work
(McDonald, 1986), the following data were presented: "Because of the
discrepant results in current and previous pregnancies a further analysis was
made of all 57 276 women employed at the start of pregnancy classified into 42
occupational groups. This was done to remove the possibility that the
recorded use of VDUs by women immediately after an abortion might not be
comparable with that by women after a full term delivery. The 42 groups were
ranked according to the percentage use of a VDU for 15 or more hours a week in
current and in previous pregnancies based on data for all women regardless of
the outcome of their pregnancies. The percentage frequencies ranged widely
from less than 5% to more than 45%. Observed to expected abortion ratios
showed no association with VDU use. In current pregnancies the ratio of
observed to expected abortions in occupations in which less than 5% of women
used a VDU for 15 or more hours a week was 1.02; with 5-24% use, 0.99 and with
45% or more use, 1.03. In previous pregnancies the ratios were as follows;

occupations with less than 5% use 0.98, 5-24% use 0.97, 25-44% use 1.03 and 45% or more use 1.02." The author concluded that: "The findings of the study give no indication that the use of a VDU in pregnancy increases the risk of congenital defect and are insufficient to reject the null hypothesis with regard to spontaneous abortion".

The Osaka Study (Kajiwara, 1984). A Japanese study on 1591 VDT-workers (789 women) included 50 pregnancies. Thirteen pregnancies were described as "abnormal pregnancies or abnormal deliveries". Of these 13 abnormal pregnancies, four (8%) ended in abortion, while six (12%) were described as threatened abortion, the remainder being "severe morning sickness" or "others". The abortion rates appear to be similar to or lower than abortion rates reported from other worker groups in Japan [e.g., for clerical workers 7.6% (Japan 1979) or 12.6% (Osaka area, 1982)]. The author did not draw any conclusions.

The National Insurance Study (Ericson et al., 1985a; 1985b). An extension of the Swedish Register study was performed. A subcohort (employees at the National Insurance) was studied, with pregnancy outcomes extended to the years 1980-1983 (miscarriages from 1980-1981 only). Data were obtained from the National Insurance as to job descriptions, and these were used to estimate the amount of VDT work for each job category. A partial validation of this estimate was possible, since 535 of the 4347 women in this study were also included in the questionnaire study made in the Swedish Register study, see below. Only 4% of these 535 women worked with VDTs more than 20 h/week.

No indications of an increased risk of miscarriage, nor for perinatal death were found. For significant malformations, 66 cases were found, compared to 69.1 expected, which gives a risk ratio of 0.96%. Specific malformations were examined, and smaller deviations were found from expected (both higher and lower). Attention was drawn primarily to a small (non-significant) excess of heart malformations (10 cases during 1981-1983, 7.2 expected). This excess was found only during 1981, and in the job categories with more VDT work.

Prior to the completion of this study, some results appeared, in which the percentages of seriously malformed children were given as 1.7, 2.3, 2.1 and 2.6

for the years 1980-1983, respectively. When Ostberg and coworkers (1985) reviewed these data, they compared them to an expected (national average) percentage of 1.7. However, the national averages were at that time not available for 1982 and 1983. When they later become available, an increase was seen in the national averages during these years as well, due to changes in registry definitions (ANON: Läkartidningen, 1985). Thus, this claim for a trend towards increased risk does not appear to be well founded.

The North Carolina Study (North Carolina Occupational Safety & Health Project, 1985). In this study, a self-reporting questionnaire was sent to 2478 persons, 40% of whom responded. Of the respondents, 966 (97%) were office workers. A part of the questionnaire concerned pregnancy outcomes of female workers or of the wives of male workers. No significant problems were detected among the survey respondents, but no details are given.

South Australia Study (Lewis et al., 1982). Within a cross-sectional study of female office workers in South Australia, a case-control substudy was performed on miscarriage rates. Of the 389 questionnaires returned, 72% were from VDT-workers with a response rate of approximately 95%. Among these, 30 of 51 reported miscarriages were selected as "cases", based on their occurrence after 1960, and being the most recent for women reporting more than one, and matched as to age and date of delivery, with 60 women as controls with normal delivery.

Of the cases, 13% had worked with VDTs while pregnant, compared to 8% among the controls. This difference was not statistically significant at the 95% confidence level. The authors concluded that "results of the case-control analysis, provided little evidence that the operation of VDUs during pregnancy is associated with an increase risk of spontaneous abortion".

The Swedish Register Study (Källén, 1985a; 1985b). In this study, conducted in Sweden by the National Board of Health and Welfare, existing registers were used to define a study group of 500 mothers with adverse pregnancy outcomes, each with two controls. In the second phase, these mothers were asked to complete a questionnaire on their work history, including use of VDTs. The response rate was 93%.

The results reviewed here will be limited to the case-control study, since only this phase of the study contained information on VDT work. The odds ratio for miscarriage was 1.1 (95% confidence interval 0.8-1.4) for VDT work (at any time during pregnancy) compared to non-VDT work. For birth defects (serious malformations and neonatal death), the corresponding odds ratio was 1.6 (1.0-2.4). Some increase in odds ratios were seen within the groups working more than 20 h/week (1.2 for spontaneous abortion, 2.3 for birth defects). The odds ratio (for all adverse outcomes) was 1.4 (1.1-1.8), but was decreased to 1.2 (0.6-2.3) when stratification for stress and smoking was performed.

The author concludes that, with due considerations to (indicated) recall bias etc., this study does not give support for the view that VDT work will cause miscarriages or significant malformations.

The Finnish Register Study (Kurppa et al., 1984; 1985). A case-control study in Finland was based on existing registers of congenital defects. A total of 1475 mothers of malformed children were included, together with paired referents (according to age, parity and other factors), and interviewed soon after delivery in the time period 1976-1982, with participation of more than 95%. These interviews covered previous pregnancies, diseases, drug consumption, etc., but not VDT work (at that time). Subsequently, two trained interviewers were involved in "exposure interviews", where the mothers were asked to give a detailed description of their work.

A number of discordant pairs (490, 235 cases and 255 referents, according to VDT work) were suggested by occupational title, 111 pairs were ascertained as to work with VDT during the first trimester by evaluation of the interview forms. In 51 discordant pairs, the VDT-worker was a "case" mother, and in 60 a "referent" mother. For VDT work, the odds ratio was 0.9 (95% confidence interval 0.6-1.3), and for VDT work more than 4 h/day (more than 20 h/week), the overall odds ratio was 1.0 (0.6-1.6). The authors conclude that "we did not detect an interdependence between VDT exposure and birth defects."

The 9 to 5 Campaign (National Association of Working Women, 1984). In this poll, 6000 questionnaires on various health aspects of VDT work were sent to callers responding to the organization's "Campaign on VDT Risks", 873 (15%)

of which were returned. Of the 216 pregnancies noted, 63 (30.6%) were
miscarriages, four (1.9%) were minor birth defects and 14 (6.8%) were major.
The authors noted the higher than normal incidence of miscarriage and major
birth defects.

Health & Safety at Work (Evans, 1985). In a second poll, a questionnaire
was printed in Health & Safety at Work, a British magazine, and also sent to
some British trade unions. The questionnaire concerned a number of health
issues including pregnancy outcome. Of the 3819 replies, 435 indicated that
they or their partners had been or were trying to become pregnant. Problems
in this respect were reported by 10% of the couples, 10% of the pregnancies
had experienced a miscarriage or a threatened miscarriage. Of the births 6%
were reported to have ended in birth defects.

An evaluation of the studies reported. There are a number of difficulties
in many of these studies. These include low response rates, e.g., 40% in the
Newspaper Guild and the North Carolina Study, and 15% in the 9 to 5 Campaign
poll. Self-administered questionnaires occur in some studies, notably in the
polls, where the questionnaire response was due to self-selection, no cohort
having been defined prior to the study.

Uncertain endpoints do occur, especially in the Health & Safety at Work
poll, where miscarriages and threatened miscarriages are combined. Definition
of birth defects are vague, e.g., in the Canadian Labour Congress Study
(1982), where the authors point out that the one recorded case of birth defect
is described as "tongue-tied". In the Health & Safety at Work poll, no
description of whether the birth defects are significant or not is given.

Many studies are also too small for valid conclusions to be made. In the
South Australia Study on 90 pregnancies, the risk ratio is 1.7, with a 95%
confidence interval of 0.10-29.04 (Lewis et al., 1982).

In evaluating these studies, the working group found that only four
studies appeared sufficiently reliable: the Montreal Study, the Finnish and
the Swedish Register Studies, and the National Insurance Study.

The working group was aware that further studies are underway in several countries, the results of which should be evaluated when available. Nevertheless, currently available data fail to provide any evidence for a link between adverse reproductive outcome and VDT work.

5.4 Recommendations for further research

The amount of work carried out on the possible health implications of working with VDTs is fairly extensive. There are however, certain areas where our knowledge is too incomplete to make a reliable assessment; these areas concern primarily stress disorders and also the possibility of skin disorders. Certain aspects of eye and muscle discomforts also need to be further studied.

Some specific areas where the working group recognized the need for further research are given below. They are not arranged in any order of priority. In such research, it is important that specific hypotheses be addressed, which are more detailed than just comparisons between VDT and non-VDT-workers.

5.4.1 Concerning effects on the eyes and vision

- A better understanding is needed of relationships between eye discomfort and specific causal or contributing factors. Such factors include various display and workroom lighting factors, aspects of job design, and also relationships between existing eye disorders and development of discomfort.

- There is also a need for longitudinal studies of visual discomforts of VDT workers.

- Further attention should also be given to occurrence of visual discomforts among some other groups of VDT workers, e.g., computer-assisted design staff and computer-assisted manufacturing operators.

5.4.2 Concerning musculoskeletal disorders

- The relationships between musculoskeletal discomfort and different tasks and job organization need further study. The influence of various patterns of rest breaks should be further investigated.

- The effects of sedentary work require further studies.

- The possibility that prolonged muscle discomfort may lead to injury or permanent damage has not been adequately addressed.

5.4.3 Concerning skin disorders

- Further epidemiological studies are needed on the possibility that skin disorders may be related to VDT work. Such studies should include the establishment for each patient of a specific diagnosis of the skin disorder.

- Possible factors that may be related to skin disorders in VDT work should be investigated. Consideration should, for example, be given exposure to ambient air pollutants in relationship to VDT work.

5.4.4 Concerning stress factors and stress disorders

- Further research should investigate specific stress factors of the VDT system, and their relation to job content and job organization. Delays and software design are two such areas of interest.

- The possible effects of different stress factors on the appearance of stress-related disorders should be further investigated. Study design should be centred on the presence of such stress factors, and not on the VDT versus non-VDT dichotomy. Some studies including objective parameters such as catecholamine excretion would be valuable.

- Further research should be performed to investigate any possible effects of the introduction of VDTs in the workplaces, especially on whether the effects that may appear are transient or permanent.

- Further research is also needed concerning the effectiveness of
strategies for the control and prevention of adverse effects appearing
during VDT work.

5.4.5 Comments

In evaluating the possible health implications of working with VDTs, the
working group noted some areas of research that are not specific for VDTs on
which further work would be warranted:

- One example is the possibility that stress factors and stress disorders
in occupational situations may be related to spontaneous abortion.

- Another example is the possible relationships between subjective eye
discomforts and objective measurements of visual or ocular functions.

- The possibility of interactions between magnetic fields and biological
systems also requires further research. This should primarily be aimed
at determining whether there are any effects of fields resembling those
found in occupational or environmental exposures. If such effects
exist, then the relevant parameters must be elucidated in order to
detect high exposure groups in occupational or nonoccupational
situations. (According to the evidence, at present available, VDT
operators do not appear to be a high exposure group.)

REFERENCES

ACGIH. TLVs, threshold limit values for chemical substances in the work environment: adopted by ACGIH for 1983-1984. Cincinnati, American Conference of Governmental Industrial Hygienists, 1983.

ANON. Coordinated effort to replicate Delgado's findings underway. Transmission/Distribution and Safety Report. 3: 1-2 (1985).

ANON. Eleventh problem pregnancy cluster reported. VDT news I, 3: 6-7 (1984).

ANON. Färre missbildade barn än väntat hos bildskärmsarbetande mödrar. [Fewer malformed children to VDT working mothers than expected.] (in Swedish). Läkartidningen, 82: 1905-1907 (1985).

ANON. NIOSH investigation: Cause of Atlanta problem pregnancy cluster unknown. VDT news II, 2: 4 (1985).

ANON. NIOSH investigating two problem pregnancy clusters. VDT news I, 2: 2-3 (1984).

ANON. VDT-pregnancy clusters prompt NIOSH research. Microwave news, 4(4) 1,12 (1984).

ARNDT, R. Working posture and musculoskeletal problems of video display terminal operators - review and reappraisal. American Industrial Hygiene Association Journal, 44: 437-446 (1983).

ARONSSON, G. Omstrukturering av kvalifikationskrav vid datorisering, [Restructuring of qualification demands during computerization.] (in Swedish). Stockholm, Institute of Psychology, University of Stockholm, (Rapporter, 1984:42).

AXELSSON, G. Miscarriage after occupational exposure: Aspects of risk assessment in retrospective studies. Göteborg, Department of Environmental Hygiene, University of Göteborg, 1983.

BACKMAN, C.M.   Lätta luftjoner i arbetsmiljö – natur, förekomst och
betydelse.   [Light air ions in working environments – nature, occurrence and
importance] (in Swedish).   University of Uppsala, UURIE, 79: 116 (1979).

BALDAUF, D.R.   The workhorse CRT: new life.   IEEE (Institute of Electrical
Electronics Engineers) Spectrum, 67-73 (July 1985).

BANBURY, J.R.   Evaluation of MTF and veiling glare characteristics for CRT
displays.   Displays, 23-29, (Jan 1982).

BAUER, D.   Causes of flicker at VDUs with bright background and ways of
eliminating interference.   In: Grandjean, E. ed.   "Ergonomics and health in
modern offices".   London, Taylor & Francis, 1984, pp. 364-370.

BAUER, D.   Reducing reflexions of external light on VDU screens – comparison
of bright and dark background screens; considerations and a case study.   In:
"Proceedings of an International Scientific Conference: Work with Display
Units".   Stockholm, 12-15 May 1986, pp. 204-205[1].

BAUER, D.   Improving the VDU workplace by introduction of a physiologically
optimized bright background screen with dark characters.   In: "Proceedings of
an International Scientific Conference: Work with Display Units".   Stockholm,
12-15 May 1986, pp. 206-207.

BAUER, D. & CAVONIUS, C.R.   Improving the legibility of visual display units
through contrast reversal.   In: Grandjean, E., Vigliani, E. eds.   "Ergonomic
aspects of visual display terminals".   London, Taylor & Francis, 1982,
pp. 137-142.

BELLUCI, R. & MAULI, F.   The effects of visual ergonomics and visual
performance upon ocular symptoms during VDT work.   In: Grandjean, E. ed.
"Ergonomics and health in modern offices".   London, Taylor & Francis, 1984,
pp. 346-351.

---

1   The Proceedings of the International Scientific Conference: Work with
    Display Units, Stockholm, 12-15 May 1986 are in preparation and their
    publication is expected early in 1987.

BENGTSSON, G. Stralskyddsinstitutets kommentar om stralning och bildskärmar. [Comments by the National Institute of Radiation Protection on radiation and VDTs.] (in Swedish). Läkartidingen, 86: 61 (1986).

BENNETT, S. & TRAPANI, G. Measurement of contrast enhancement in VDU screens. Displays, 167-170 (July 1983).

BENOIT, F.M., LEBEL, G.L., WILLIAMS, D.T. Are video display terminals a source of increased PCB concentration in the working atmosphere? One answer. International archives of occupational and environmental health, 53: 261-267 (1984).

BERGQVIST, U.OV. Video display terminals and health. Scandinavian journal of work, environment & health, 10 (suppl 2): 1-87 (1984).

BERGQVIST, U., WIBOM, R. & NYLEN, P. Electrostatic fields at VDT work stations - a review. In: "Proceedings of an International Scientific Conference: Work with Display Units". Stockholm, 12-15 May 1986, pp. 45-48.

BINASCHI, S. ET AL. Study on subjective symptomatology of fatigue in VDU operators. In: Grandjean, E. & Vigliani, E. eds. "Ergonomic aspects of visual display terminals". London, Taylor & Francis, 1982, pp. 219-225.

BINKIN, N.J., ROCHAT, R.W., CATES, W., TYLER, C.W. Cluster of spontaneous abortion, Dallas, Texas. Atlanta, Center for Disease Control, Public Health Service, 1981. (Unpublished memorandum EPI-80-113-2).

BINNIE, C.D., KASTELEIJN-NOLST TRENITE, D.G.A., DE KORTE, R., WILKINS, A. Visual display units and risk of seizures. Lancet, i: 991 (1985).

BJORSET, H.E., & BREKKE, B. The concept of contrast. A short note and a proposal. In: Grandjean, E., Vigliani, E., eds. "Ergonomic aspects of visual display terminals". London, Taylor & Francis, 1982, pp. 23-24.

BJORSETH, A., WARNCKE, M., URSIN, H. Stress hos gravide: Konsekvenser for mor og barn [Stress in pregnant women: consequences for mother and child] (in Norwegian). Borgen Dept. of Physiological Psychology, University of Bergen, 1985.

BOLINDER, G. (1983). Dataterminalarbete vid Karolinska Sjukhuset. [VDT work at the Karolinska Hospital.] (in Swedish). Solna, National Board of Occupational Safety and Health, 1983. (Work project FLAK II 1981/1983).

BOOS, S.R., ET AL. Work at video display terminals. An epidemiological health investigation of office employees. III. Ophthalmological examination. Scandinavian journal of work, environment & health, 11: 475-481 (1985).

BOUMA, H. Visual reading processes and the quality of text displays. In: Grandjean, E, Vigliani, E. eds. "Ergonomic aspects of visual display terminals". London, Taylor & Francis, 1982, pp. 101-114.

BRAUNINGER, U., GRANDJEAN, E., GUERER, R., FELLMANN, T. Lighting characteristics of visual display terminals of different makes. Ergonomics, 25: 556 (1982).

BROWN, C.R. & SCHAUM, D.L. User-adjusted VDU parameters. In: Grandjean, E., Vigliani, E., eds. "Ergonomic aspects of visual display terminals". London, Taylor & Francis, 1982, pp. 195-200.

BUREAU OF RADIOLOGICAL HEALTH. An evaluation of radiation emission from video display terminals. Rockville, Health and Human Services, Publication FDA 81-8153, 1981.

CAKIR, A., HART, D.J., STEWART, T.F.M. The VDT manual. Darmstadt, International Federation of Newspaper Publishers - International Research Association for Newspaper Technology (INCA-FIEJ), 1980.

CAMPBELL, F.W. & DURDENT, K. The visual display terminal issue: A consideration of its physiological, psychological and clinical background. Ophthalmic physiology and optics, 3: 175-192 (1983).

CANADIAN LABOUR CONGRESS Towards a more humanized technology; exploring the impact of Video Display Terminals on the health and working conditions of Canadian office workers, Ottawa, Labour Education and Studies Centre, 1982.

CATO OLSEN, W. Electric field enhanced aerosol exposure in visual display unit environments. Bergen, Charles Michelsen Institute, 1981 (CMI 803604-1).

CATO OLSEN, W. Facial exposure in the VDU environment: The role of static electricity. In: "Proceedings of an International Scientific Conference: Work with Display Units". Stockholm, 12-15 May 1986, pp. 797-800.

CHARRY, J.M. DC Electric fields, air ions and respirable particulate levels in proximity to VDTs. Presented at the International Scientific Conference: "Work with Display Units". Stockholm, 12-15 May 1986.

COMMONWEALTH DEPARTMENT OF HEALTH. Repetition strain injury in the Australian Public Service. Task Force Report. Canberra, Australian Government Publishing Service, July 1985.

CORNO, F. & DENIEUL, P. Analysis of small disturbances of accommodation related to visual display units. In: "Proceedings of an International Scientific Conference: Work with Display Units". Stockholm, 12-15 May 1986, pp. 948-951.

COX, E.A. Radiation emission from visual display units. In: Pearce, B.G. ed. "Health hazards of VDTs?" Chichester, Wiley, 1984, pp. 25-37.

DAINOFF, M.J. Visual fatigue in VDT-operators. In: Grandjean, E. & Vigliani, E. eds. "Ergonomic aspects of visual display terminals". London, Taylor & Francis, 1982a, pp. 95-99.

DAINOFF, M.J. Occupational stress factors in visual display terminals (VDT) operation: A review of empirical research. Behaviour and information technology, 1: 141-176 (1982b).

DAINOFF, M.J., HAPP, A., CRANE, P. Visual fatigue and occupational stress in VDT-operators. Human factors, 23: 421-438 (1981).

DATADELEGATIONEN. Framtida bildskärmar. [Future VDTs] (in Swedish). Stockholm, Civildepartementet, DS.C. 21: 1985.

DE GROOT, J.P. & KAMPHUIS, A. Eyestrain in VDU users: Physical correlates and long-term effects. Human factors, 25: 409-413 (1983).

DELGADO, J.M.R. Electromagnetic effects: From insects to humans.
In: "Proceedings of a Symposium on Biomagnetism in Psychophysiology,
1st International Conference on Psychophysiology", Montreal,
August 1982.

DELGADO, J.M.R., LEAL, J., MONTEAGUDO, J.L., GRACIA, M.G. Embryological
changes induced by weak, extremely low frequency electromagnetic fields.
Journal of anatomy, 134: 533-551 (1982).

DELVOLE, N. & QUEINNEC, Y. Operator's activities at CRT terminals: a
behavioural approach. Ergonomics, 26: 329-340 (1983).

DEMATTEO, B. The hazards of VDTs. 2nd ed. Toronto, Ontario Public Service
Employees Union, 1984.

DIGERNES, V. & ASTRUP, E.G. Are datascreen terminals a source of increased
PCB-concentrations in the working atmosphere? International archives of
occupational and environmental health, 49: 193-197 (1982).

EHRLICH, D. Transient myopia following sustained near work. In: "Proceedings
of an International Scientific Conference: Work with Display Units".
Stockholm, 12-15 May 1986, pp. 956-959.

ELIAS, R., CAIL, F., TISSERAND, M., CHRISTMANN, H. Investigations in
operators working with CRT display terminals: relationships between task
content and psychophysiological alterations. In: Grandjean, E., Vigliani, E.
eds. "Ergonomic aspects of visual display terminals". London, Taylor &
Francis, 1982, pp. 211-217.

ELINSON, L., ROSENBAUM, L., HANCOCK, T., CAPLAN, G. Health effects of video
display terminals. Toronto, Health Advocacy Unit, Department of Public
Health, 1980.

ENGEL, F.L. Information selection from visual display unit. In: Grandjean,
E., Vigliani, E. eds. "Ergonomic aspects of visual display terminals".
London, Taylor & Francis, 1982, pp. 121-125.

ERICSON, A., KALLEN, B., WESTERHOLM, P. Graviditetsutfall bland kvinnor, anställda under gravididet vid den allmänna försäkringskassan i Sverige 1980-1983. [Pregnancy outcome among women, employed during pregnancy by the National Insurance in Sweden, 1980-1983.] (in Swedish). Stockholm, National Board of Health and Welfare, 1985a.

ERICSON, A., KALLEN, B., WESTERHOLM, P. Ingen ökad risk för fosterskador hos kvinnor med bildskärmsarbete. [No increased risk of birth defects among women with VDT work.] (in Swedish). Läkartidningen, 82: 2180-2184 (1985b).

ERIKSSON, S. Temporal and spatial stability in visual displays. In: "Proceedings of an International Scientific Conference: Work with Display Units". Stockholm, 12-15 May 1986, pp. 380-382.

ECMA Ergonomics - recommendations for VDU work places. Zürich, European Computer Manufacturers Association, 1984 (ECMA/TR/22).

EVANS, J. VDU operators display health problems. Health and safety at work, 33-37 (November 1985).

EVANS, J. Questionnaire survey of British VDU operators. In: "Proceedings of an International Scientific Conference: Work with Display Units". Stockholm, 12-15 May 1986, pp. 565-568.

FARRELL, J.E. & MORAN, M.A. A method for predicting screen flicker. In: "Proceedings of an International Scientific Conference: Work with Display Units". Stockholm, 12-15 May 1986, pp. 372-375.

FELLMANN, Th., BRAUNINGER, U., GIERER, R., GRANDJEAN, E. An ergonomic evaluation of VDTs. Behaviour and information technology, 1: 69-80 (1982).

FERGUSON, D. The "new" industrial epidemic. Medical journal of Australia, 17 March 1984, 318-319.

FLORU, R. & CAIL, F. Data entry task on VDU: Underload or overload? In: "Proceedings of an International Scientific Conference: Work with Display Units". Stockholm, 12-15 May 1986, pp. 265-268.

FRANK, A.L. Effects on health following occupational exposure to video display terminals. Lexington, Department of Preventive Medicine and Environmental Health, University of Kentucky, 1984 (40536-0084).

GALITZ, W.O. Screen design. In: Grandjean, E. ed. "Ergonomics and health in modern offices". London, Taylor & Francis, 1984, pp. 400-404.

GHINGIRELLI, L. Collection of subjective opinions on use of VDUs. In: Grandjean, E., Vigliani, E. eds. "Ergonomic aspects of visual display terminals". London, Taylor & Francis, 1982, pp. 227-231.

GOULD, J.D. & GRISCHKOWSKY, N. Doing the same work with hard copy and with cathode-ray tube (CRT) computer terminals. Human factors, 26: 323-337 (1984).

GRAF, W., SIGL, F., VAN DER HAIDEN, G. & KRUEGER, H. The applicability of eye movement analysis in the ergonomic evaluation of human-computer interaction. In: "Proceedings of an International Scientific Conference: Work with Display Units". Stockholm, 12-15 May 1986, pp. 512-515.

GRANDJEAN, E. Ergonomics and medical aspects of VDU workplaces. Displays, 76-80, July 1980.

GRANDJEAN, E., HUNTING, W., NISHIYAMA, K. Preferred VDT workstation settings, body posture and physical impairments. Applied ergonomics, 15: 99-104 (1984).

GREENWALD, M.J., GREENWALD S.L., BLAKE, R. Long-lasting visual aftereffect from viewing a computer video display. New England journal of medicine, 309: 315 (1983).

GRIECO, A., MOLTENI, G., PICCOLI, B. Field study in newspaper printing: a systematic approach to VDU operator strain. In: Grandjean, E. & Vigliani, E. eds. "Ergonomic aspects of visual display terminals". London, Taylor & Francis, 1982, pp. 185-194.

GRIGNOLO, F.M., et al. Considerations on ocular motility and refractive errors in VDU operators. In: Grandjean, E. ed. "Ergonomics and health in modern offices". London, Taylor & Francis, 1984, pp. 431-435.

GRIGNOLO, F.M., DI BARI, A., BROGLIATTI, N., PALUMBO, A., MAINA, G. Ocular tonometry in VDU operators. In: "Proceedings of an International Scientific Conference: Work with Display Units". Stockholm, 12-15 May 1986, pp. 578-581.

GRIVET, P. Electron optics. 2nd Ed. Oxford, Pergamon Press, 1972, pp. 380-426.

GUEKOS, G. & ULMI, R. Room illumination and CRT/flicker in visual display terminals. CIE journal, 2: 6-11 (1983).

GUNNARSSON, E. & SODERBERG, I. Arbete vid textskärmar pa tidningsföretag. [Work at text display units in newspapers.] (in Swedish), Undersökningsrapport, 21, 1979 (National Board of Occupational Safety and Health, Solna, Sweden).

GUNNARSSON, E. & SODERBERG, I. Eye strain resulting from VDT work at the Swedish Telecommunications Administration. Applied ergonomics, 14: 61-69 (1983).

GUY, A.W. Non-ionizing radiation: Dosimetry and interaction. In: "Non-Ionizing Radiation, Proceedings of a Topical Symposium, 26-28 Nov 1979, Washington DC", American Conference of Governmental Industrial Hygienists, 1980.

GUY, A.W. Health hazards assessment of radio frequency electromagnetic fields emitted by video display terminals. Report prepared for IBM Office of the Director of Health and Safety, Corporate Headquarters, Armonk, 2 December 1984.

HAGBERG, M., SUNDELIN. G., HAMMARSTRÖM, U. Belastning pa skulder-nack muskel vid ordbehandlingsarbete med bildskärm. [Static load on shoulder-neck muscle during work with VDT word processor] (in Swedish). 34 Nordiske yrkeshygieniska mötet, Tampere, 1-3 October 1985, 48-49.

HAIDER, M., KUNDI, M., WEISSENBÖCK, M. Worker strain related to VDUs with differently coloured characters. In: Grandjean, E. & Vigliani, E. eds. "Ergonomic aspects of visual display terminals". London, Taylor & Francis, 1982, pp. 53-64.

HARVEY, S.M. Electric-field exposure of persons using video display units. Bioelectromagnetics, 5: 1-12 (1984).

HAUBNER, P. & KOKOSCHKA, S. Visual display units - characteristics of performance. 20th Session of the Commission internationale d'éclairage (CIE) 1983, B3. Amsterdam, International Commission on Illumination, 1983.

HAUBNER, P. & BENZ, C. Information display on monochrome and colour screens. In: Grandjean, E. ed. "Ergonomics and health in modern offices". London, Taylor & Francis, 1984, pp. 371-376.

HEDMAN, L. Ackommodations- och konvergensförändringar hos expeditörer med bildskärmsarbete. [Accommodation and convergence changes in VDU workers.] (in Swedish). Farsta, Televerkets arbetsmiljösektion, 1982 (Rapport 1982:01).

HEDMAN, L.R. & BRIEM, V. Short-term changes in eyestrain of VDU users as a function of age. Human factors, 26: 357-370 (1984).

HERON, R.M. VDT ergonomics and the question of job design: Implications for women. Presented at the "Conference on Women and the Impact of Microtechnology, Ottawa, 25 June 1982".

HERRING, V. & BERNS, T. Literature review. Positive vs negative image polarity of visual display screens. Stockholm, Ergolab, 1984.

HIRNING, C.R. & AITKEN J.H. Cathode-ray tube X-ray emission standards for video display terminals. Health physics, 43: 727-731 (1982).

HOWARTH, P.A. & ISTANCE, H.O. The association between visual discomfort and the use of visual display units. Behaviour information technology, 4: 131-149 (1985).

HUGHES, D. Hazards of occupational exposure to ultraviolet radiation. Northwood, Science Reviews. Occupational hygiene monograph, No. 1, reprint, 1982a.

HUGHES, D. Notes on ionizing radiation: Quantities, units, biological effects and permissible doses. Northwood, Science Reviews. Occupational hygiene monograph, No. 5, 1982b.

HüNTING, W., LäUBLI, T., GRANDJEAN, E. Postural and visual loads at VDT workplaces I. Constrained postures. Ergonomics, 24: 917-931 (1981).

IBM. Human factors of workstations with visual displays, 3rd Ed. San José, Human Factors Center, 1984.

Institut de recherche en santé et en sécurité du travail du Québec, (1983). Work and pregnancy: Outline protocol and progress, Nov. 1981 - Nov. 1983. Quebec.

Institut de recherche en santé et en sécurité du travail du Québec. Report of the Task Force on Video Display Terminals and Workers' Health S-0003, Montreal, May 1984.

ILO/WHO. Report of the Joint ILO/WHO Committee on Occupational Health, Ninth Session, on Recognition and Control of Adverse Psycho-Social Factors at Work, JCOH/1984/D.6(rev), Geneva, International Labour Office, 18-24 September 1984.

ISENSEE, S.H. & BENNETT, C.A. The perception of flicker and glare on computer CRT displays. Human factors, 25: 177-184 (1983).

IWASAKI, T. & KURIMOTO, S. Measurements of vergent eye movement by jumping method before and after VDT work. Acta ophtalmologica, Suppl 164, 24 (1984).

IWASAKI, T. & KURIMOTO, S. Influence of visible and invisible flicker on "floating accommodation". In: "Proceedings of an International Scientific Conference: Work with Display Units". Stockholm, 12-15 May 1986, pp. 387-390.

JARVINEN, E. & MAKITIE, J. VDU work: Refractive errors and binocular vision. In: "Proceedings of an International Scientific Conference: Work with Display Units". Stockholm, 12-15 May 1986, pp. 136-138.

JASCHINSKI-KRUZA, W. Transient myopia after visual work. Ergonomics, 27: 1181-1189 (1984).

JASCHINKSI-KRUZA, W. Is the resting state of our eyes a favourable viewing distance for VDU work? In: "Proceedings of an International Scientific Conference: Work with Display Units". Stockholm, 12-15 May 1986, pp. 952-955.

JEAVONS, P.M. et al. Visual display units and epilepsy. Lancet, i: 287 (1985).

JOHANSSON, G. Growth and challenge vs wear and tear of humans in computer mediated work. In: "Proceedings of an International Scientific Conference: Work with Display Units". Stockholm, 12-15 May 1986, pp. 249-251.

JOHANSSON, G. & ARONSSON, G. Stress reactions in computerized administrative work. Journal of occupational behaviour, 5: 159-181 (1984).

JOHNSON, B.L. & MELIUS, J.M. A review of NIOSH's VDT studies and recommendations. In: "Proceedings of an International Scientific Conference: Work with Display Units". Stockholm, 12-15 May 1986, pp. 481-484.

JUUTILAINEN, J. & SAALI, K. Effects of low frequency magnetic fields on the development of chick embryos. In: "Proceedings of an International Scientific Conference: Work with Display Units". Stockholm, 12-15 May 1986, pp. 71-72.

JUUTILAINEN, J., HARRI, M., SAALI, K., LAHTINEN, T. Effects of 100-Hz magnetic fields with various waveforms on the development of chick embryos. Radiation and environmental biophysics, (in press) (1986).

KAJIWARA, S. Work and health in VDT workplaces. (in Japanese.) Osaka, In-Service Training Institute for Safety and Health of Labour, 1984, pp. 5-82.

KALLEN, B. En epidemiologisk studie över arbete med dataskärm och graviditet. [An epidemiological study of VDT work and pregnancy.] (in Swedish). Lund, Department of Embryology, University of Lund, 1985a.

KALLEN, B. Dataskärmsarbete och graviditet [VDT work and pregnancy.] (in Swedish). Läkartidningen, 82: 1339-1342 (1985b).

KALSBEK, J.W.H. & UMBACH, F.W. Tasks involving contrast resolution, spatial and temporal resolution presented on VDU screens as a measuring technique of visual fatigue. In: Grandjean, E., Vigliani, E. eds. "Ergonomic aspects of visual display terminals". London, Taylor & Francis, 1982, pp. 71-76.

KEMMLERT, K., KILBOM, A., MILERAD, E., WISTEDT, C. <u>Musculo-skeletal trouble in the neck and shoulders - relationship with clinical findings and workplace design in offices</u>. In: "Proceedings of an International Scientific Conference: Work with Display Units". Stockholm, 12-15 May 1986, pp. 174-177.

KESSEL, K.L. <u>Task analysis in applying software design principles</u>. In: Grandjean, E. ed. "Ergonomics and health in modern offices". London, Taylor & Francis, 1984, pp. 170-174.

KHAN, J.A., FITZ, J., PSALTIS, P., IDE, C.H. Prolonged complementary chromatopsia in users of video display terminals. <u>American journal of ophthalmology</u>, <u>98</u>: 756-758 (1984).

KILBOM, A. <u>Physiological effects of extreme physical inactivity - a brief review</u>. In: "Proceedings of an International Scientific Conference: Work with Display Units". Stockholm, 12-15 May 1986, pp. 486-489.

KLIGMAN, A.M. Early destructive effects of sunlight on human skin. <u>Journal of the American Medical Association</u>, <u>210</u>: 2377-2380 (1969).

KNAVE, B.G. et al. Work at video display terminals. An epidemiological health investigation of office employees. I. Subjective symptoms and discomforts. <u>Scandinavian journal of work, environment & health</u>, <u>11</u>: 457-466 (1985a).

KNAVE, B.G. et al. Work at video display terminals. An epidemiological health investigation of office employees. II. Physical exposure factors. <u>Scandinavian journal of work, environment & health</u>, <u>11</u>: 467-474 (1985b).

KNILL-JONES, R.P. <u>Adverse pregnancy outcome amongst lady doctors - lessons from twelve years of research</u>. In: "Proceedings of an International Meeting to Examine the Allegations of Reproductive Hazards from VDUs". London, 29-30 November 1984, pp. 177-185.

KNUTSSON, A. <u>Computerization in industry causes problems for people with reading and writing difficulties (dyslexia)</u>. In: "Proceedings of an International Scientific Conference: Work with Display Units". Stockholm, 12-15 May 1986, pp. 366-367.

KOKOSCHKA, S. A method for optimizing the character contrast of CRT-displays. In: "Proceedings of an International Scientific Conference: Work with Display Units". Stockholm, 12-15 May 1986, pp. 280-284.

KROEMER, K.H.E. & HILL, S.G. Preferred line of sight. In: "Proceedings of an International Scientific Conference: Work with Display Units". Stockholm, 12-15 May 1986, pp. 415-418.

KUHNE, A., KRUEGER, H., GRAF, W., MERZ, L. Positive versus negative image polarity. In: "Proceedings of an International Scientific Conference: Work with Display Units". Stockholm, 12-15 May 1986, pp. 208-211.

KUMASHIRO, M. A mechanism of mental stress response on VDT performance. In: Grandjean, E. ed. "Ergonomics and health in modern offices". London, Taylor & Francis, 1984, pp. 240-247.

KURIMATO, S. ET AL. Influence of VDT work on eye accommodation. Journal of UOEH University of Occupational and Environmental Health, 5: 101-110, (1983).

KURPPA, K., HOLMBERG, P.C., RANTALA, K., NURMINEN, T. Birth defects and video display terminals. Lancet, ii: 8, 1339 (1984).

KURPPA, K. ET AL. Birth defects and exposure to video display terminals during pregnancy. Scandinavian journal of work, environment & health, 11: 353-356 (1985).

LABOUR CANADA. In the chips: Opportunities - people - partnerships. Ottawa, Task Force on Micro-Electronics and Employment, 1982.

LAGERHOLM, B. Bildskärmar och hudförändringar: Ingaende undersökningar motiverade. [VDTs and skin changes: Close investigations motivated.] (in Swedish). Läkartidningen, 83: 60-61 (1986).

LANDRIGAN, P.J. ET AL. Reproductive hazards in the workplace. Scandinavian journal of work, environment & health, 9: 83-86 (1983).

LAUBLI, T., HUNTING, W., GRANDJEAN, E. Postural and visual loads at VDT workplaces. II. Lighting conditions and visual impairments. Ergonomics, 24: 933-944 (1981).

LAUBLI, T. Review on working conditions and postural discomforts in VDT work.
In: "Proceedings of an International Scientific Conference: Work with Display
Units". Stockholm, 12-15 May 1986, pp. 3-6.

LAVILLE, A. Postural reactions related to activities in VDU. In: Grandjean,
E., Vigliani, E. eds. "Ergonomic aspects of visual display terminals".
London, Taylor & Francis, 1982, pp. 167-174.

LEE, B.V. & McNAMEE, R. Reproduction and work with visual display units - a
pilot study. In: "Proceedings of an International Meeting to Examine the
Allegations of Reproductive Hazards from VDUs". London, 29-30 November 1984,
pp. 41-47.

LERMAN, S. Radiant energy and the eye. Vol. 1. New York, Macmillan, 1980
(Functional ophthalmology series).

LEVY, F. & RAMBERG, I.G. Eye fatigue among VDU users and non-VDU users. In:
"Proceedings of an International Scientific Conference: Work with Display
Units". Stockholm, 12-15 May 1986, pp. 631-634.

LEWIS, M.J., ESTERMAN, A.J., DORSCH, M.M. A survey of the health consequences
to females of operating visual display units. Community health studies, 6:
130-134 (1982).

LIDEN, C. & WAHLBERG, J.E. Work at video display terminals. An epidemiological
health investigation of office employees. V. Dermatological examination.
Scandinavian journal of work, environment & health, 11: 489-493 (1985a).

LIDEN, C. & WAHLBERG, J.E. Does visual display terminal work provoke rosacea?
Contact dermatitis, 12: 235-241 (1985b).

LIDEN, C. & WAHLBERG, J.E. VDT work and skin. In: "Proceedings of an
International Scientific Conference: Work with Display Units". Stockholm,
12-15 May 1986, pp. 801-802.

LINDEN, C. & ROLFSEN, S. Video computer terminals and occupational dermatitis.
Scandinavian journal of work, environment & health, 7: 62-63 (1981).

LOFGREN, B. Ortopedmedicinsk undersökning av skulder-nack-besvär vid bildskärmsarbete. [Medical examination of discomfort in shoulders and neck during VDT work.] (in Swedish). Solna, National Baord of Occupational Safety and Health, 1985, (FLAK 84/85).

MacKAY, C. Visual display unit operation: possible reproductive effects. In: "Proceedings of an International Meeting to Examine the Allegations of Reproductive Hazards from VDUs". London, 29-30 November 1984, pp. 137-159.

MacKAY, C. & COX, T. Occupational stress associated with visual display unit operation. In: Pearce, B.G. "Health hazard of VDTs?" Chichester, Wiley, 1984, pp. 137-143.

MAFFEO, S., MILLER, L.W., CARSTENSEN, E.L. Lack of effect of weak low-frequency magnetic fields on chick embryogenesis. Journal of anatomy, 139: 613-618 (1984).

MANDAL, A.C. The influence of furniture height on backpain. In: "Proceedings of an International Scientific Conference: Work with Display Units". Stockholm, 12-15 May 1986, pp. 427-430.

MAREK, T. & NOWOROL, C. Mental fatigue of VDU operators induced by monotonous and various tasks. In: "Proceedings of an International Scientific Conference: Work with Display Units". Stockholm, 12-15 May 1986, pp. 261-264.

MARRIOTT, I.A. & STUCHLY, M.A. Health aspects of work with video display terminals. Working paper at a "Review Meeting on Health Impact of VDTs". Geneva, World Health Organization, 21-23 May 1985.

McDONALD, A.D. Epidemiology of spontaneous abortions, birth defects and prematurity. In: "Proceedings of an International Meeting to Examine the Allegations of Reproductive Hazards from VDUs". London, 29-30 November 1984, pp. 5-26.

McDONALD, A.D. Birth defect, spontaneous abortion and work with VDUs. In: "Proceedings of an International Scientific Conference: Work with Display Units". Stockholm, 12-15 May 1986, pp. 669-670.

McDONALD, A.D. ET AL. Work and pregnancy in Montreal - Preliminary findings. Presented at the "Third Conference on Epidemiology in Occupational Health", Singapore, 28-30 September 1983.

McDONALD, A.D., CHERRY, N.M., DELORME, C., McDONALD, J.C. Work and pregnancy in Montreal - Preliminary findings on work with visual display terminals. In: "Proceedings of an International Meeting to Examine the Allegations of Reproductive Hazards from VDUs". London, 29-30 November 1984, pp. 161-175.

McPHEE, B. Occupational cervicobrachial disorders in VDT users. In: Proceedings of an International Scientific Conference: Work with Display Units. Stockholm, 12-15 May 1986, pp. 163-166.

MELLNER, M. & MOBERG, I. Belastnings- och synbesvär vid arbete med dataterminal [Visual and muscular discomforts during VDT work.] (in Swedish). Stockholm, Oxens Företagshälsovard, 1983.

MEYER, J.J. et al. Sensitivity to light and visual strain of VDU operators. "Proceedings of the IVth World Congress of Ergoophthalmology". Naples, 26-30 May 1985.

MEYER, J.J., REY, P., SCHIRA, J.-C., BOUSQUET, A. Sensitivity to light and visual strain in VDT operators: Basic data for the design of work stations. In: "Proceedings of an International Scientific Conference: Work with Display Units". Stockholm, 12-15 May 1986, pp. 289-293.

MIKOLAJCZYK, H., INDULSKI, J., PAWLACZYK, M., WALICKA, L., BIENKOWSKA-JANUSZKO, E. Miscarriages in pregnant women employed at VDU and effects of TV radiation on experimental animals. In: "Proceedings of an International Scientific Conference: Work with Display Units". Stockholm, 12-15 May 1986, pp. 64-67.

MILLAR, J.D. Statement before the Subcommittee on Health and Safety, Committee on Education and Labor, House of Representatives, Washington DC, 1984.

MILLAR, W. & SUTHER, T.W. Display station anthropometrics: Preferred height and angle settings of CRT and keyboard. Human factors, 25: 401-408 (1983).

MOHANNA, S., SHERMAN, G.J., STUCHLY, M.A. Review of the report by Sharma, H.D. (1984) (g.v.) Ontario, Canadian Radiation Protection Bureau, 1986.

MOSS, C.E., MURRAY, W.E., PARR, W.H., MESSITE, J. KARSHES, G.J. A report on electromagnetic radiation survey of video display terminals. Cincinnati, Public Health Service, 1977, NIOSH Technical Report 78-129.

MOURANT, R.R., LAKSHMANAN, R., CHANTADISAI, R. Visual fatigue and cathode ray tube display terminals. Human factors, 23: 520-540 (1981).

MURCH, G.M. & BEATON, R.J. Matching display characteristics to human visual capacity. In: "Proceedings of an International Scientific Conference: Work with Display Units". Stockholm, 12-15 May 1986, pp. 452-455.

MURRAY, W.E., MOSS, C.E., PARR, W.H., COX, C. A radiation and industrial hygiene survey of video display terminal operations. Human factors, 23: 413-420 (1981a).

MURRAY, W.E. ET AL. Potential health hazards of video display terminals. Cincinnati, Public Health Service, 1981b. (NIOSH Research Report 81-129).

NATIONAL ASSOCIATION OF WORKING WOMEN. 9 to 5 Compaign on VDT risks hotline. Cleveland, 1983.

NATIONAL ASSOCIATION OF WORKING WOMEN. 9 to 5 Campaign on VDT risks. Analysis of VDT operator questionnaire of VDT hotline callers, Cleveland, 1984.

NBOSH. Buller i arbetslivet. Anvisning 110/1976 [Noise during work provision.] (in Swedish), Solna, National Board of Occupational Safety and Health, Sweden, 1976.

NBOSH. Infraljud och ultraljud i arbetslivet. Anvisning 110:1/1978. [Infra- and ultrasound at work provision.] (in Swedish), Solna, National Board of Occupational Safety and Health, Sweden, 1978.

NBOSH. Högfrekventa elektromagnetiska fält, förslag. [High frequency electromagnetic fields, proposal.] (in Swedish). Solna, National Board of Occupational Safety and Health, Sweden, 1985a.

NBOSH. <u>Arbete vid bildskärm</u>. AFS 1985:12. [Work with video display units.] (in Swedish), Solna, National Board of Occupational Safety and Health, Sweden, 1985b.

NBOSH. <u>Electromagnetic radiation and fields at visual display terminals</u> <u>(VDTs)</u>. Solna, National Board of Occupational Safety and Health, Sweden, 1986.

NATIONAL OCCUPATIONAL HEALTH AND SAFETY COMMISSION. <u>Interim report of the</u> <u>Repetition Strain Injury Committee</u>. Canberra, Australian Government Publishing Service, July 1985.

NATIONAL RESEARCH COUNCIL, PANEL ON IMPACT OF VIDEO VIEWING ON VISION OF WORKERS. <u>Video displays, work and vision</u>. Washington DC, National Academy Press, 1983.

NILSEN, A. Facial rash in visual display unit operators. <u>Contact dermatitis</u>, <u>8</u>: 25-28 (1982).

NISHIYAMA, K. ET AL. Physiological effects of oscillating luminances in reversed display of VDTs. <u>Ergonomics</u>, <u>25</u>: 555-556 (1982).

NISHIYAMA, K., NAKASEKO, M., UEHATA, T. <u>Health aspects of VDT operators in</u> <u>the newspaper industry</u>. In: Grandjean, E. ed. "Ergonomics and health in modern offices". London, Taylor & Francis, 1984, pp. 113-118.

NORTH CAROLINA OCCUPATIONAL SAFETY AND HEALTH PROJECT. <u>Stress survey</u> <u>results</u>. Durham, March 1985.

NYLEN, P. <u>Non-elevated levels of polychlorinated biphenyls in two offices</u> <u>with VDTs and fluorescent lighting</u>. Oslo, 33 Nordiske yrkeshygieniske möte, 8-10 October 1984, pp. 18-19.

NYLEN, P. A light phenomenon perceived when viewing CRT-based VDT screens with positive image. <u>Applied ergonomics</u>, <u>16</u>: 82-84 (1985).

NYLEN, P. & BERGQVIST, U. <u>Visual phenomena and their relation to top</u> <u>luminance, phosphor persistence time and contrast polarity</u>. In: "Proceedings

of an International Scientific Conference: Work with Display Units".
Stockholm, 12-15 May 1986, pp. 285-288.

NYLEN, P., BERGQVIST, U., WIBOM, R., KNAVE, B. Physical and chemical
environment at VDT work stations. "Proceedings of the 3rd International
Conference on Indoor Air Quality and Climate", Stockholm, 20-24 August 1984.

NYMAN, K.G., KNAVE, B.G., VOSS, M. Work at video display terminals. An
epidemiological health investigation of office employees. IV. Studies on
refraction, accommodation, convergence and binocular vision during work.
Scandinavian journal of work, environment & health, 11: 483-487 (1985).

ONG, C.-N. & PHOON, W.-O. Influence of age on VDU work. In: "Proceedings of
an International Scientific Conference: Work with Display Units". Stockholm,
12-15 May 1986, pp. 17-20.

ONG, C.N., HOONG, B.T., PHOON, W.O. Visual and muscular fatigue in operators
using visual display terminals. Journal of human ergology, 1: 161-171 (1981).

OSTBERG, O. Accommodation and visual fatigue in display work. Displays,
81-85 (July 1980).

OSTBERG, O., AHLSTROM, G., MOLLER, L. Ergonomic procurement guidelines for
visual display units as a tool for progressive change. In: "Proceedings of
the Eleventh International Symposium on Human Factors in Telecommunication",
Cesson-Sévigné, 9-13 September 1985.

PADMOS, P. & POT, F. Determinants of the VDU operator's well-being. 1.
Visual and postural ergonomics, optometry. In: "Proceedings of an
International Scientific Conference: Work with Display Units". Stockholm,
12-15 May 1986, pp. 167-170.

PAULSSON, L.E., KRISTIANSSON, I., MALMSTROM, I. Stralning fran data-skärmar,
arbetsdokument a 84-08 [Radiation from VDTs.] (in Swedish) Stockholm, Statens
Stralskyddsinstitut, 1984.

PAULSSON, L.E. Radiation emissions from VDUs. In: "Proceedings of an International Scientific Conference: Work with Display Units". Stockholm, 12-15 May 1986, pp. 25-28.

PHILLIPS, B.G. Video display terminals. An Alberta view. Presented at the Second General Meeting of the Canadian Radiation Protection Association, Ottawa, May 1981.

PITTS, D.G., CULLEN, A.P., DAYHAW-BARKER, P. Determination of ocular thresholds levels for infrared radiation cataractogenesis. Cincinnati, Public Health Service, 1980 (NIOSH Research Report 80-121).

POMROY, C. & NOEL, L. Low-background radiation measurements on video display terminals. Health physics, 46: 413-417 (1984).

POT, F., BROUWERS, A., PADMOS, P. Determinants of the VDU operator's well-being. 2. Work organization. In: "Proceedings of an International Scientific Conference: Work with Display Units". Stockholm, 12-15 May 1986, pp. 322-324.

PURDHAM, J. Adverse pregnancy outcome amongst VDT-operators - the cluster phenomenon. In: "Proceedings of an International Meeting to Examine the Allegations of Reproductive Hazards from VDUs". London, 29-30 November 1984, pp. 27-40.

RADL, G.W. Experimental investigations for optimal presentation-mode and colours of symbols on the CRT-screen. In: Grandjean, E., Vigliani, E. eds. "Ergonomic aspects of visual display terminals". London, Taylor & Francis, 1982, pp. 127-135.

REPACHOLI, M.H. Video display terminals - should operators be concerned? Adelaide, University of Adelaide (In press).

REY, P. & MEYER, J.J. Visual impairments and their objective correlates. In: Grandjean, E. & Vigliani, E. eds. "Ergonomic aspects of visual display terminals". London, Taylor & Francis, 1982, pp. 77-83.

REY, P., MEYER, J.J., BOUSQUET, A. Surveillance médicale des opérateurs sur écran cathodique. Klin. Mbl. Augenheilk., 180: 370-372 (1982).

ROGOWITZ, B. <u>Measuring perceived flicker on visual displays</u>. In: Grandjean, E. ed. "Ergonomics and health in modern offices". London, Taylor & Francis, 1984, pp. 285-293.

ROMANO, C. & SONNINO, A. <u>Efficiency of data entry by VDUs. A comparison between different softwares</u>. In: Grandjean, E. ed. "Egronomics and health in modern offices". London, Taylor & Francis, 1984, pp. 187-191.

ROSENBAUM, L. Health effects of video display terminals. The nonradiation problems. Toronto, Health Advocacy Unit, Department of Public Health, 1981.

ROWE, S., OXENBURGH, M., DOUGLAS, D. <u>Repetition strain injury amongst keyboard operators in a large Sydney office</u>. In: "Proceedings of an International Scientific Conference: Work with Display Units". Stockholm, 12-15 May 1986, pp. 635-638.

ROWLAND, J.B. <u>Health complaints associated with video display terminals among telephone operators</u>. Presented at the "Conference on Impact of Office Automation and Computermediated Work on the Quality of Work Life". 10-12 December 1984, Washington DC, US Congress, Office of Technology Assessment.

RUBINO, G.F., ET AL. <u>Visual impairment and subjective ocular symptomatology in VDU operators</u>. In: "Proceedings of an International Scientific Conference: Work with Display Units". Stockholm, 12-15 May 1986, pp. 697-700.

RYCROFT, R.J.G. & CALNAN, C.D. <u>Facial rashes among visual display unit (VDU) operators</u>. In. Pearce, B.G, ed. "Health hazards of VDTs?" Chichester, Wiley, 1984, pp. 13-15.

SANDELL, J., MAKITIE, J., LEHTELA, J. <u>Ergonomic evaluation of multifocal lenses in work with visual display units</u>. In: "Proceedings of an International Scientific Conference: Work with Display Units". Stockholm, 12-15 May 1986, pp. 134-135.

SANDSTROM, M., HANSSON MILD, K., LOVSTRUP, S. <u>Effects of weak pulsed magnetic fields on chick embryogenesis</u>. In: "Proceedings of an International Scientific Conference: Work with Display Units". Stockholm, 12-15 May 1986, pp. 60-63.

SARRA, A. Ocular motility and binocular coordination recorded "in situ" at VDU screen. In: "Proceedings of an International Scientific Conference: Work with Display Units". Stockholm, 12-15 May 1986, pp. 142-144.

SAUTER, S. Predictors of strain in VDT users and traditional office workers. In: Grandjean, E. et. "Ergonomics and health in modern offices". London, Taylor & Francis, 1984, pp. 129-135.

SAUTER, S.L. ET AL. Job and health implications of VDT use: Initial results of the Wisconsin-NIOSH Study. Communications of the ACM, 26: 285-294 (1983a).

SAUTER, S.L., GOTTLIEB, M.S., ROHRER, K.M., DODSON, V.N. The well-being of video display terminal users. An exploratory study. Madison, University of Wisconsin, Department of Preventive Medicine, 1983b (210-79-0034).

SAUTER, S.L., CHAPMAN, L.J., KNUTSON, S.J., ANDERSON, H.A. Wrist trauma in VDT keyboard use: Evidence, mechanisms and implications for keyboard and wrist rest design. In: "Proceedings of an International Scientific Conference: Work with Display Units". Stockholm, 12-15 May 1986, pp. 230-234.

SAUTER, S.L., ET AL. Chronic neck-shoulder discomfort in VDT use: Prevalence and medical observations. In: "Proceedings of an International Scientific Conference: Work with Display Units". Stockholm, 12-15 May 1986, pp. 154-158.

SAXEN, L. Epidemiological studies for detection of teratogens. In: Infante, P.F. & Legator, M.S. eds. "Proceedings of a workshop on methodology for assessing reproductive hazards in the workplace, 19-22 April 1978". Cincinnati, Public Health Service, pp. 357-404 (NIOSH 81-100).

SCHLEIFER, L.M. Effects of VDT/computer system response delays and incentive pay on mood disturbances and somatic discomfort. In: "Proceedings of an International Scientific Conference: Work with Display Units". Stockholm, 12-15 May 1986, pp. 447-450.

SCHULDT, K., EKHOLM, J., HARMS-RINGDAHL, K. Sitting work postures and movements, and muscular activity in neck and shoulder muscles. In: "Proceedings of an International Scientific Conference: Work with Display Units". Stockholm, 12-15 May 1986, pp. 338-340.

SELL, R.G. Quality of working life and the introduction of new technology into the office. In: Grandjean, E. ed. "Ergonomics and health in modern offices". London, Taylor & Francis, 1984, pp. 160-164.

SERRA, A. Far point of VDU operators measured in situ. In: Grandjean, E. ed. "Ergonomics and health in modern offices". London, Taylor & Francis, 1984, pp. 260-264.

SHAHNAVAZ, H. Lighting conditions and workplace dimensions of VDU-operators. Ergonomics, 25: 1165-1173 (1982).

SHAHNAVAZ, H. & HEDMAN, L.R. Visual accommodation changes in VDU operators related to environmental lighting and screen quality. Ergonomics, 27: 1071-1082 (1984).

SHARMA, H.D. The investigation of a cluster of adverse pregnancy outcomes and other health-related problems among employees working with video display terminals in the accounting office at the Surrey Memorial Hospital, Vancouver, B.C., Waterloo, REMS, 1984.

SHUTE, S.J. & STARR, S.J. Effects of adjustable furniture on VDT users. Human factors, 26: 157-170 (1984).

SIVAK, J.G. & WOO, G.C. Color of visual display terminals and the eye. Green VDTs provide the optimal stimulus to accommodation. American journal of optometric physiology and optics, 60: 640-642 (1983).

SMITH, A.B., TANAKA, S., HALPERIN, W., RICHARDS, R.D. Report of a cross-sectional survey of video display terminal (VDT) users at the Baltimore Sun. Cincinnati, National Institute for Occupational Safety and Health, Centers for Disease Control, September 1982.

SMITH, A.B., TANAKA, S., HALPERIN, W. Correlates of ocular and somatic symptoms among video display terminal users. Human factors, 26: 143-156 (1984).

SMITH, M.J. Health issues in VDT work. Cincinnati, Motivation and Stress Research Section, National Institute for Occupational Safety and Health, 1982.

SMITH, M.J., COHEN, B.G.F., STAMMERJOHN, L.W. An investigation of health complaints and job stress in video display operations. Human factors, 23: 387-400 (1981).

SMITH, M.J., STAMMERJOHN, L.W., COHEN, B.G.F., LALICH, N.R. Job stress in video display operations. In: Grandjean, E. & Vigliani, E. eds. "Ergonomics aspects of visual display terminals". London, Taylor & Francis, 1982, pp. 101-210.

SMITH, W. Computer color: Psychophysics, task application, and aesthetics. In: "Proceedings of an International Scientific Conference: Work with Display Units". Stockholm, 12-15 May 1986, pp. 561-564.

STAMMERJOHN, L.W., SMITH, M.J., COHEN, B.G.F. Evaluation of work station design factors in VDT-operations. Human factors, 23: 401-412 (1981).

STANDARDISERINGSKOMMISSIONEN I SVERIGE, (1983). Ergonomics - Requirements in visual information processing - Image quality on cathode ray tube (CRT) based visual display units (VDU) for text presentation in office environments. Stockholm. (Draft 2 1983-06-06).

STARR, S.J. A study of video display terminal workers. Journal of occupational medicine, 25: 95-98 (1983).

STARR, S.J. Effects of video display terminals in a business office. Human factors, 26: 347-356 (1984).

STARR, S.J., THOMPSON, C.R., SHUTE, S.J. Effects of video display terminals on telephone operators. Human factors, 24: 699-711 (1982).

STELLMAN, J.M., KLITZMAN, S., GORDON, G.R., SNOW, B. Comparison of well-being among full-time, part-time VDT users, typists and non-machine interactive clerical workers. In: "Proceedings of an International Scientific Conference: Work with Display Units". Stockholm, 12-15 May 1986, pp. 303-306.

STENBERG, B. An outbreak of a rosacea-like skin rash in VDU-operators. In: "Proceedings of an International Scientific Conference: Work with Display Units". Stockholm, 12-15 May 1986, p. 803.

STUCHLY, M.A., LECUYER, D.W., MANN, R.D. Extremely low frequency electromagnetic emissions from video display terminals and other devices. Health physics, 45: 713-722 (1983a).

STUCHLY, M.A., REPACHOLI, M.H., LECUYER, D.W., MANN, R.D. Radiofrequency emissions from video display terminals. Health physics, 45: 772-775 (1983b).

SUNDGREN, P.E. Större material maste utnyttjas vid forskning om graviditetsrisker. [Larger populations must be used in research on pregnancy risks.] (in Swedish). Läkartidningen, 82: 2490-2492 (1985).

TAKAHASHI, M., IIDA, H., NISHIOKA, A., KUBOTA, S. An appropriate luminance of VDT characters. In: Grandjean, E. ed. "Ergonomics and health in modern offices". London, Taylor & Francis, 1984, pp. 316-321.

TARRANT, A.W.S., BROWNS, S., LAYCOCK, J. Research Note. Measured and perceived colour on cathode ray tubes. Displays, 162-166 (July 1983).

TAYLOR, S.E. & McVEY, B.W. The dynamics of dark focus and accommodation to dark and light character CRT displays. In: Grandjean, E. ed. "Ergonomics and health in modern offices". London, Taylor & Francis, 1984, pp. 248-253.

TERRANA, T., MERLUZZI, F., GIUDICI, E. Electromagnetic radiations emitted by visual display units. In: Grandjean, E., Vigliani, E. eds. "Ergonomic aspects of visual display terminals". London, Taylor and Francis, 1982, pp. 13-21.

TIMMERS, H., VAN NES, F.L., BLOMMAERT, F.J.J. Visual work recognition as a function of contrast. In: Grandjean, E., Vigliani, E. eds: "Ergonomic aspects of visual display terminals". London, Taylors & Francis, 1982, pp. 115-120.

TJONN, H.H. Report of facial rashes among VDU operators in Norway. In: Pearce, B.G. ed. "Health hazards of VDTs?" Chichester, Wiley, 1984, pp. 17-23.

TRAVERS, H.P. & STANTON, B.A. Office workers and video display terminals: Physical, psychological and ergonomic factors. Occupational health nursing, 32: 586-591 (1984).

TRIBUTAIT, B., CEKAN, E., PAULSSON, L-E. Effects of pulsed magnetic fields on embryonic development in mice. In: "Proceedings of an International Scientific Conference: Work with Display Units". Stockholm, 12-15 May 1986, pp. 68-70.

TRILLO, M.A. et al. Alterations and fractional recovery of chick embryos exposed to electromagnetic fields. In: "Third Annual Meeting of the Bio-electrical Repair Society, San Fransisco, 2-5 October 1983". (Abstract).

TURNER, P.J. Visual requirements for VDU operators. Australian journal of optometry, 65: 58-64 (1982). (Additional details in Coe, J.B. et al., Visual display units. Wellington, New Zealand Department of Health, 1980, Report W/1/180).

UBEDA, A. ET AL. Pulse shape of magnetic fields influences chick embryogenesis. Journal of anatomy, 137: 513-536 (1983).

UNGETHUM, E. Elektriska fält i närheten av dataskärmar och dess beydelse för transport av luftburen fororening. [Electrical fields in the vicinity of VDTs and their importance for transport of air contaminants.] (in Swedish). Oslo, 33 Nordiske yrkeshygieniske möte, 8-10 October 1984, p. 17.

UNIVERSITY OF PARK PRESS. Airborne particles, medical and biologic effects of environmental pollutants. Baltimore, University of Park Press, 1979.

USSR Standard for Occupational Exposure GOST 12.1.006-76 (with supplement 1/1984 [Admissable limit level according to electrical compounds (E-field)], and USSR Standard for Occcupational Exposure 12.1.045-84 (1984) [Electrostatic fields. Admissable rates at workplaces and requirements to control procedures] Moskva, Izdaletstvo Slandartor (in Russian).

VAN DER HEIDEN, G.H., BRAUNINGER, U., GRANDJEAN, E. Ergonomic studies on computer aided design. In: Grandjean, E. ed. "Ergonomics and health in modern offices". London, Taylor & Francis, 1984, pp. 119-128.

VAN NES, F.L.   Colour on displays - boon or curse?   In: "Proceedings of an International Scientific Conference: Work with Display Units".   Stockholm, 12-15 May 1986, pp. 628-630.

VERRIEST, G., ANDREW, I., UVILJS, A.   Study of visual performance on a multi-color VDU of color-defective and normal trichromatic subjects.   In: "Proceedings of an International Scientific Conference: Work with Display Units".   Stockholm, 12-15 May 1986, pp. 368-371.

VON KIPARSKI, R.   Experiences of routine technical measurement analysis of VDT working places in the field of occupational health service.   In: Grandjean, E. ed.   "Ergonomics and health in modern offices".   London, Taylor & Francis, 1984, pp. 136-140.

WAERN, Y. & ROLLENHAGEN, C.   Reading text from visual display units (VDUs).   International journal of man-machine studies, 18: 441-465 (1983).

WALLACH, C.   Effects of cathode ray video displays on human health.   Presented at the "Fourth Annual Meeting of the Bio-electromagnetics Society",   Los Angeles, June 1982.

WALLIN, L., WINKVIST, E., SVENSSON, G.   Terminalanvändares arbetsmiljö - en enkätstudie vid Volvo i Göteborg.   [The work environment of terminal users - a questionnaire study at Volvo in Gothenburg.]   (in Swedish),   Gothenburg, AB Volvo, 1983.

WALSH, M.L. & FACEY, R.A.   Synopsis of the phase I report of project HAVDU (Hazard assessment of video display terminals).   Pickering, Health and Safety Division, November 1983.

WARR, A.   Operating VDUs.   Work organisation and subjective effects on operator health and psychology.   Journal of physiological ergonomics and scientific instrumentation, 14: 530-540 (1981).

WEISS, M.M.   The video display terminals - Is there a radiation hazard?   Journal of occupational medicine, 25: 98-101 (1983).

WEISS, M.M. & PETERSEN, R.C. Electromagnetic radiation emitted from video computer terminals. <u>American Industrial Hygiene Association Journal</u>, <u>40</u>: 300-309 (1979).

WENNBERG, A. & VOSS, M. <u>Videocoding - a highly monotonous VDU work in a new technique for mail sorting</u>. In: "Proceedings of an International Scientific Conference: Work with Display Units". Stockholm, 12-15 May 1986, pp. 270-273.

WESTINGHOUSE. <u>Phosphor guide for industrial and military cathode-ray tubes</u>. Elmira, Westinghouse, 1972.

WESTLANDER, G. <u>Occupational factors affecting stress</u>. Solna, National Board of Occupational Safety and Health, Work Psychology Unit, 1984.

WESTLANDER, G. <u>Kontorsarbete som objekt för arbetsmiljöforskning,</u> undersökningsrapport 1985:6 [Office work as a target for work environment research.] (in Swedish). Solna, National Board of Occupational Safety and Health, Sweden, 1985.

WESTLANDER, G. <u>How identify organizational factors crucial of VDU-health?</u> In: "Proceedings of an International Scientific Conference: Work with Display Units". Stockholm, 12-15 May 1986, pp. 80-85.

WHO. <u>Ultraviolet radiation</u>. Geneva, World Health Organization, 1979 (Environmental Health Criteria 14).

WHO. <u>Radiofrequency and microwaves</u>. Geneva, World Health Organization, 1981 (Environmental Health Criteria 16).

WHO. <u>Extremely low frequency (ELF) fields</u>. Geneva, World Health Organization, 1984 (Environmental Health Criteria 35).

WICHANSKY, A.M. <u>Legibility and user acceptance of monochrome display phosphor colors</u>. In: "Proceedings of an International Scientific Conference: Work with Display Units". Stockholm, 12-15 May 1986, pp. 216-219.

WINKEL, J. Macro-and micro-circulatory changes during prolonged sedentary work and the need for lower limit values for leg activity - a review. In: "Proceedings of an International Scientific Conference: Work with Display Units". Stockholm, 12-15 May 1986, pp. 497-500.

WILKINS, A.J. ET AL. Television epilepsy - the role of pattern. Electroencephalographic and clinical neurophysiology, 47: 163-171 (1979).

WILKINS, R. VDTs in the workplace: Problems and prospects. Montreal, Institute for Research on Public Policy, 1983.

WOLBARSHT, M.L. ET AL. Electromagnetic emission from visual display units. A non-hazard. In: "Non-ionizing radiation, Proceedings of a Topical Symposium, 26-28 Nov 1979, Washington DC". Cincinnati, American Conference of Governmental Industrial Hygienists, 1980, pp. 193-200.

WOO, G.C., STRONG, G., IRVING, E., ING., B. Are there subtle changes in vision after use of VDTs? In: "Proceedings of an International Scientific Conference: Work with Display Units". Stockholm, 12-15 May 1986, pp. 875-877.

WRIGHT, I. Identification and prevention of work-related mental and psychosomatic disorders among two categories of VDU users. In: "Proceedings of an International Scientific Conference: Work with Display Units". Stockholm, 12-15 May 1986, pp. 308-130.

WU, S.S.-H., ET AL. Blink rate as a measure of effort in visual task performance. In: "Proceedings of an International Scientific Conference: Work with Display Units". Stockholm, 12-15 May 1986, pp. 705-712.

YAMAMOTO, S. & NORO, K. Characterization of VDT work. In: "Proceedings of an International Scientific Conference: Work with Display Units". Stockholm, 12-15 May 1986, pp. 94-96.

YAMAMOTO, S., NORO, S., KURIMOTO, S. & IWASAKI, Y. VDT operators' variation of the accommodation of the eyes during VDT work. In: "Proceedings of an International Scientific Conference: Work with Display Units". Stockholm, 12-15 May 1986, pp. 878-881.

ZARET, M. <u>Cataracts following use of cathode ray tube displays</u>. Presented at the "Symposium UPSI sur Ondes Electromagnetique et Biologie" Jouy-en-Josas, July 1980.

ZARET, M. <u>Cataracts and visual display units</u>. In: Pearce, B.G. ed. "Health hazards of VDTs?" Chichester, Wiley, 1984, pp. 47-54.

ZEIER, H., ET AL. <u>Psychophysiological correlates between postural discomfort, personality, and muscle tension</u>. In: "Proceedings of an International Scientific Conference: Work with Display Units". Stockholm, 12-15 May 1986, pp. 159-162.

ZUK, W.M., STUCHLY, M.A., DVORAK, P., DESLAURIERS, Y. <u>Investigation of radiation emissions from video display terminals</u>. Ottawa, Radiation Protection Bureau, Health and Welfare of Canada (83-EHD-91).

ZULCH, J., KRUEGER, H. & HAITZ, P. <u>Fourier analytical approximation of the flicker quality of CRTs</u>. In: "Proceedings of an International Scientific Conference: Work with Display Units". Stockholm, 12-15 May 1986, pp. 376-379.

ZWAHLEN, H.T. & HARTMANN, A.L. <u>VDT operator pupil diameter changes, accommodation changes and subjective comfort/discomfort score changes over a working day</u>. "Proceeding of the Human Factors Society: 29th Annual Meeting", 1985, pp. 630-634.

ZWAHLEN, H.T. & KOTHARI, N. <u>The effects of dark and light character CRT displays upon VDT operators performance, eye scanning behaviour, pupil diameter and subjective comfort/discomfort</u>. In: "Proceedings of an International Scientific Conference: Work with Display Units". Stockholm, 12-15 May 1986, pp. 220-223.

LIST OF PARTICIPANTS IN THE WHO WORKING GROUP ON
OCCUPATIONAL HEALTH ASPECTS IN THE USE OF VISUAL DISPLAY TERMINALS

Geneva, 2-6 December 1985

Members

Dr S.E. Asogwa, Department of Community Medicine, College of Medicine,
University of Nigeria, Enugu, Nigeria

Dr Ulf OV. Bergqvist, Research Department, National Board of Occupational
Safety and Health, Solna, Sweden (Rapporteur)

Dr Ahmed Emara, Department of Occupational Medicine, Faculty of Medicine,
Cairo Universty, Kasr-el-Eini, Cairo, Egypt

Professor Bengt G. Knave,[1] Research Department, National Board of
Occupational Safety and Health, Solna, Sweden

Professor A.O. Navakatikian, Kiev Research Institute of Labour Hygiene and
Occupational Diseases, Kiev, USSR

Professor Paule Rey, University of Geneva, Department of Occupational Medicine
and Ergonomics, Geneva, Switzerland

Dr Steven Sauter, Division of Biomedical and Behavioural Sciences, National
Institute for Occupational Safety and Health, Cincinnati, Ohio, USA (Chairman)

Dr T.F.M. Stewart, Systems Concepts Ltd, Museum House, Museum Street, London,
England

---

1 Also represented the International Ergonomics Association

Representatives of other organizations

International Labour Office

Dr J. Stellman,[1] Occupational Safety and Health Branch, Working Conditions
and Environment Department, ILO, Geneva, Switzerland

International Federation of Commercial, Clerical, Professional and Technical
Employees (FIET)

Mr. Guy Ryder, Geneva, Switzerland

Secretariat

Dr M.A. El Batawi, Chief Medical Officer, Office of Occupational Health, WHO,
Geneva, Switzerland

Dr T. Ng, Medical Officer, Office of Occupational Health, WHO, Geneva,
Switzerland

Dr C. Xintaras, Scientist, Office of Occupational Health, WHO, Geneva,
Switzerland (Secretary)

_____

1 Unable to participate.

VISUAL DISPLAY TERMINALS OF NON-CATHODE RAY TUBE DESIGN

Construction principles

Visual display terminals can be based on techniques other than
conventional cathode ray tubes (CRTs). These techniques are primarily based
on plasma displays, electroluminescense or liquid crystal displays. VDTs
using these techniques are available on the market. Brief discussions of
these techniques are to be found in (Andersson, 1983; Apt, 1985; Daae, 1985;
Hamnerius, 1986; Lagebrand, 1983 and Perry, 1985). The most important
difference between these techniques and the conventional CRT technique is in
the addressing function, since all rely on some sort of physical matrix.

Plasma displays (PD) utilize a thin gas layer (e.g. neon or argon), which
can be ionized by a current. This current is delivered by conductors, and
ionization and thus visible discharge occurs only at the junction of two live
conductors in a matrix (see Fig. 1). The choice of gas determines the colour
- orange with neon.

Electroluminescent displays (ELD) are constructed with a thin phosphor
layer (fluorescent screen material) that reacts to a sufficiently strong
electric field (e.g. an AC field at 16 kHz). These fields appear at the
junction of horizontal and vertical conductors, placed at opposite sides of
the layer.

Liquid crystal display (LCD) techniques are also being developed. In
LCDs, light is refracted in liquid crystals, whose refractive capability is
determined by an electric field: in contrast to the other techniques, LCD
screens do not emit any light, but are dependent on incoming light, which put
additional restraints on office lighting. In a picture element, transmission
of this light is then determined by the electric field in the 'junction'
(determining whether the element will be 'dark' or 'bright').

Considerable efforts are being made to develop these techniques further,
in order to improve the visual presentation, increase the size of the screen,

and decrease the production costs. Additional designs, e.g. light emitting
diodes (LEDs), or combining CRT techniques with plasma (Anon., 1983) or with
a current multiplier (Mansell et al., 1983) are also being developed.
Considerable improvements have also been made in conventional CRT techniques
(see Baldauf, 1985).

Advantages and disadvantages of these new techniques

These new VDT techniques have both advantages and disadvantages compared to
conventional CRTs. Some problems are inherent in the design while others are
probably soluble by further development. These problems concern visual
characteristics such as resolution, contrast, luminance variation, etc. One
major obstacle is the principle of 'matrix addressing', which involves a
matrix of individual cells (pixels) at the intersections of a maze as in
Fig. 1. Some of the lines in the matrix carry current, depending on the
information to be displayed. The improvement of resolution, by the
construction of more cells, may be more costly with these techniques than with
conventional CRTs.

In the following discussion, based on papers by Andersson (1983), Apt
(1985), Daae (1985), Datadelegation (1985), Lagebrand (1983), Perry (1985),
Werner (1985), and Ny Teknik (1985), advantages and disadvantages are referred
to only when they concern factors involved, or probably involved, in the
appearance of adverse health effects. Furthermore, the following list of
advantages and disadvantages are based on observations of designs at present
available and may thus not necessarily apply to other designs being
developed. Some studies are underway to further assess the ergonomic factors
related to these techniques.

Fig. 1.   "MATRIX" SYSTEM USED IN SEVERAL TYPES OF NON-CRT-BASED VDTs

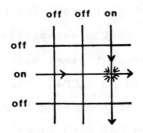

<u>Advantages</u>: The major advantages of these 'new' techniques compared to conventional CRT techniques are:

- flat displays, thus less cumbersome to place in an office, with more flexibility as to position, which could lead to easier design of ergonomically appropriate workstations (flat panel CRTs are also being developed);
- low weight;
- stable presentation because there is no variation of light emission with time – thus no tendency to flicker (this does not at present apply to LCDs, where the crystal configuration must be 'refreshed'; in PDs, there is a 16 kHz signal – but this is not detectable by the eye);
- no jitter or edge distortion.

<u>Disadvantages</u>: There are, however, several ergonomic disadvantages of these screen techniques:

- constrast is too low (especially LCD and PD);
- luminance is too low, and there is no possibility of regulating the luminance (PD and ELD);
- character structure is not optimal (ELD and LCD);
- picture elements (pixels) are often not dots but, for example, discrete and discontinuous circles or ellipses (PD);
- small size of screen (hitherto true of ELD and LCD, but larger screens are now appearing on the market);
- slow changes during information renewal (LCD);
- difficulty when viewing the screen from an oblique angle (LCD);
- increased dependence on office lighting (LCD);
- difficulty in presenting several colours (PD) or use of a (fixed) suboptimal colour (orange in neon PD);
- limited resolution because of the matrix construction – the problem of resolution and the difficulty of providing multicolour presentation, may be the major obstacles to the acceptance of these techniques. Werner (1985), gives the present pixel size as 0.07 mm (CRTs), 0.05 mm (ELD), 0.25 mm (PD) and 0.10 mm (LCD). It has been claimed (Hansson G, personal communication), that improving these parameters will be more difficult with non-CRT than CRT techniques (for fundamental reasons).

Apt (1985) made an evaluation of image quality of these four techniques (see Annex 2 Table 1). In the Table 'numerical grades' have been assigned to the descriptive terms used by Apt (for example, poor = 1; fair = 2; good = 3, and excellent = 4). The totals of the 'numerical grades' are as follows: CRT = 28.5, ELD = 21.5, LCD = 15.5 and PD = 21 (32 = excellent on all points, 8 = poor on all points). These numerical assessments of image quality are in accordance with the general view that the CRT techniques are at present superior as regards image quality compared to the other techniques, and that LCDs have the poorest image quality (see Paci & Ormezzano, 1986 or Perry, 1985).

Annex 2 Table 1. Image quality of different VDT techniques[a]

Parameter	Cathode ray tube (CRT)	Electrolumine- scent display (ELD)	Liquid crystal display (LCD)	Plasma display (PD)
Brightness	4	4	2 – 3	4
Resolution	3 – 4	3	2 – 3	3
Contrast	3 – 4	3	2	3
Gray scale	4	2	1	1
Viewing angle	4	3	1	3 – 4
Colour capability	4	1	1	1
Image stability	2	4	3 – 4	4
Motion targeting	3 – 4	1 – 2	2	1 – 2

[a] Modified from Apt (1985). 1 = poor, 2 = fair, 3 = good, 4 = excellent.
[Numerical grades by the reviewers. Further considerations can be given to
the relative importance of each parameter and to the numerical value given
each grade assigned by Bergqvist. However, the overall evaluation of
these techniques (CRT being better than ELD, and PD than LCD) is not
changed by reasonable numerical readjustments).]

In addition to these factors, the small magnitude of low frequency magnetic
fields and ultrasound, and low electrostatic fields have been used to
encourage acceptance of these techniques. However, in the absence of
indications of any effect of these factors, it seems improper to give weight
to the relative absence of a magnetic field against suboptimal visual
ergonomics.

It should be noted, that no comprehensive study has been made, evaluating
the ergonomic impact on operators using VDTs based on these techniques. The
ergonomic factors noted in the preliminary list above were chosen on the basis
of experience from CRT-based VDTs. Further discussion on this is found in a
report by the US National Research Council (1983).

REFERENCES

ANDERSSON, P.A. Smektisk LCD ger tunn bildskärm [Smectic LCD gives flat
display.], Elteknik med elektronik 6:86-89 (1983) (in Swedish).

ANON. Flat terminal combines plasma and CRT techniques. Displays, 172-173,
(July 1983).

APT, C.M. Perfecting the picture. IEEE Spectrum, July 1985, 60-66.

BALDAUF, D.R. The workhorse CRT: new life. IEEE Spectrum, July 1985, 67-73.

Bildskärmarna: Alternativen är dyrare och sämre [VDTs: Alternatives are more
expensive and worse] Ny Teknik, 18 (1985) (in Swedish.).

DAAE, K.I. Arbeidsplasser med dataterminaler. Ergonomi, syns og
belysningsforhold. Dataterminaler teknisk oversikt. Framtida muligheter.
[VDT workplaces. Ergonomics, visual and lighting conditions. Technical
review, future possibilities]. Oslo, Norwegian Institute of Technology, 9-11
January 1985 (in Norwegian).

DATADELEGATIONEN. Framtida bildskärmar. [Future VDTs]. Swedish Civil
departmentet DSC 21: (1985) (in Swedish).

HAMNERIUS, Y. Flat panel displays - alternative to CRT. In: "Proceedings of
an International Scientific Conference: Work with Display Units". Stockholm,
12-15 May 1986, pp. 902-905.

LAGEBRAND, L. Den tunna platta bildskärmen är här. [The thin flat display is
here]. Industriell Datateknik, 4:68-69 (1983) (in Swedish).

MANSELL, J.R. ET AL. The metal-dynode mutliplier: a new component in CRT
design. Displays, 135-139 (July 1983).

NATIONAL RESEARCH COUNCIL, PANEL ON IMPACT OF VIDEO VIEWING ON VISION OF
WORKERS. Video display, work and vision. Washington, DC. National Academy
Press, 1983.

PACI, A.M. & ORMEZZANO, V. <u>A comparative ergonomic evaluation of CRT displays</u> <u>and other emerging technologies</u>. In: "Proceedings of an International Scientific Conference: Work with Display Units". Stockholm, 12-15 May 1986, pp. 465-468.

PERRY, T.S. From lab to lap. <u>IEEE Spectrum</u>, 53-59, July 1985.

WERNER G. Förstudie - jämförande produkttestning av data-bildskärmar [Pilot study - comparative testing of VDTs]. Boras, Statens Provningsanstalt, SP-RAPP, 3, 1985 (in Swedish).

A MODEL STUDY ON THE OCCURRENCE OF ADVERSE PREGNANCY OUTCOMES IN CLUSTERS OF WORKERS USING VISUAL DISPLAY TERMINALS[1]

Definition of the problem

A number of groups of VDT-operators have been found, for which the rates of spontaneous abortion and congenital defects were considerably higher than for the normal population. These findings should be evaluated as to possible explanations - chance, work-related factors, or nonwork-related factors. In this appendix the possibility of a chance explanation will be examined.

The findings could be due to a combination of (i) chance (the random accumulation of a number of adverse pregnancy outcome cases in a few small groups out of a large number of groups) and (ii) selection bias (the reporting of only these groups with high rates, without normal or subnormal rates in other groups being reported). This suggestion was investigated in a model by the computation of the expected number of groups with a rate of spontaneous abortion of 50% (or a rate of congenital defects of 35%) on the assumption that the rate of spontaneous abortions or congenital defects among all VDT-workers was the same as that of the general population (null hypothesis).

Model assumptions

Some simplifying assumptions had to be made. The three described variables (population size, group size, and adverse outcome rates) were assigned reasonably well-motivated values for the calculations. Variations in all variables were then made within justifiable limits.

---

1 The text is taken from U.OV. Bergqvist, "Video display terminals and health", in the Scandinavian journal of work, environment & health, 10 (suppl 12): 80-82 (1984).

Model population. The estimated number of VDT-operators in the USA (7 000 000 in 1981, according to an unpublished memorandum of Binkin et al.) includes more than 50% women. In this memorandum, Binkin and coworkers used a pregnancy rate of 20 out of 92 workers during three years for estimates, based on data from the Sears-Roebuck cluster (see Table 4., page 139). The use of similar pregnancy rate (7% per year) would mean about 500 000 pregnant women working with VDTs during 1981 in the USA.

A pregnancy rate of about 5% was used in the model, the result being an estimate of 350 000 pregnant VDT-operators per year, to be used in the calculations. This value, which is not expected to be wrong by more than a factor of two in either direction, was used for the present model study only.

These 350 000 pregnant women were then divided into 29 200 groups with twelve pregnant women in each (spontaneous abortion model), and 35 000 groups with ten pregnant women in each (congenital defect model).

Rates of adverse pregnancy outcomes. The rate of spontaneous abortion was assumed to be 12.6% (mean of reported data in the study of Axelson (1983), with a range of 8.9 to 15.3%). Binkin and coworkers, in their unpublished memorandum, used 14.4% as the rate for their estimates, whereas McDonald et al. (1983) reported a rate of 18.1%.

Rates of congenital defects appear to be less well defined; rates of between 1.3 and 4.5% were found in the literature (Elinson et al., 1980; McDonald et al., 1983; Saxén, 1980). The rate used for the model calculation was 2%.

Spontaneous abortion

The probability distribution of the number of spontaneous abortions in the groups is hypergeometrical (no return), i.e. Hyp (350 000, 12, 0.126), which can be approximated with a binomial distribution, Bin (12, 0.126).

In Fig. 1 the expected number of groups per year with a rate of spontaneous abortion higher than x is shown as a function of x. As can be seen, close to 5400 of the 29 200 groups should be expected to have a spontaneous abortion rate higher than twice the normal rate. The model suggests that 55 groups would be expected to have a rate of spontaneous abortion higher than 50%. (During 1979-1980 (one year), six groups were reported with a mean spontaneous abortion rate of 52%).

Variations in the assumptions. Variations in group size and miscarriage rate are shown in Table 1. Most combination results show that some groups should be expected to have at least a 50% miscarriage rate. Only in the case of the largest group size used (N=20) and the smallest miscarriage rate found in the literature (8.9%), should no group be expected to have a miscarriage rate exceeding 50%. However, this does not necessarily imply that the result (in this combination) is a statistically significant deviation from the null hypothesis.

The size of the total population will affect the results only proportionally. If the population size is doubled, the number of expected groups will also be doubled. Increases in the total model population size occur for (i) the inclusion of Canadian data and (ii) an extension of the (model) study time period.

Conclusion. The appearance of six groups of high rates of spontaneous abortions which have been reported in Canada and the USA during one year (in 1979-1980) is consistent with the hypothesis, that the rate of spontaneous abortion among VDT-operators is the same as in the general population.

Congenital defects

The probability distribution of the number of congenital defects in the groups of the model is hypergeometrical, ie. Hyp (350 000, 10, 0.02), which can be approximated with a binomial distribution, Bin (10, 0.02).

The expected number of groups per year with a rate of congenital defects higher than x is shown as a function of x in Fig. 1. Approximately 6400 of 35 000 groups should be expected to have a rate of congenital defects higher than 10%. Six groups are expected to have a rate higher than 35%. During 1979-1980 (one year) three groups were reported with a mean rate of congenital defects of about 35%.

Variations in the assumptions. Variations in group size and rate of congenital defects are shown in Table 2. The majority of the combinations shows that some groups should be expected to have at least a 35% congenital defect rate. Assumption of a small rate among the total population (1.3%) indicates that the group size is crucial. The failure in some combinations to show that the reported numbers agree or are lower than the expected numbers do not suggest that the deviation is statistically significant. The previous comments made on the total population size are valid also for these calculations.

Conclusion. The three groups of high rates of congenital defects which have been reported in Canada and the USA during 1979-1980 agree reasonably well with the estimates on the expected number of groups that should appear, according to the model. Thus, chance appears to be a plausible explanation of these findings.

REFERENCES

AXELSSON, G. Miscarriage after occupational exposure: aspects of risk assessment in retrospective studies. Department of Environmental Hygiene, University of Göteborg, Göteborg, Sweden, 1983.

ELISON, L. ET AL. Health effects of video display terminals. Health Advocacy Unit, Department of Public Health, Toronto, Ontario, 1980.

McDONALD, A.D. ET AL. Work and pregnancy in Montreal - Preliminary findings. Presented at the Third Conference on Epidemiology in Occupational Health, Singapore, 28-30 September 1983.

SAXÉN, L. Epidemiological studies for detection of teratogens. In: Infante P.F., Legator M.S., eds. Proceedings of a workshop on methodology for assessing reproductive hazards in the workplace, 19-22 April 1978. Cincinnati, Public Health Service, 1980, pp. 357-404 (NIOSH 81-100).

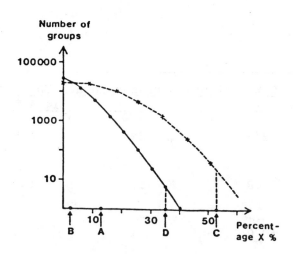

Fig. 1. The expected number of groups per year with a frequency of adverse
pregnancy higher than x % as a function of x. The rate of spontaneous
abortion used for the calculations was 12.6%, and the group size was 12 –
total of 29 200 groups. The rate of congenital defects used for the
calculations was 2.0 %, and the group size was 10 – total of 35 000 groups.
(A = normal rate of spontaneous abortions used for the calculations, B =
normal rate of congenital defects used for the calculations, C = observed rate
of spontaneous abortions in six reported clusters in one year (1979–1980), D =
observed rate of congenital defects in three reported clusters in one year
(1979–1980), x----x = spontaneous abortions, •————• = congenital defects.)

Annex 3 Table 1.   Calculated number of groups which will be expected to have a frequency of miscarriage higher than 50 %, with variations due to different assumptions.

Assumed group sizes[1]	Rates of miscarriages in all VDT-exposed pregnancies			
	8.9 %	12.6 %	14.4 %	18.1 %
7 (50 000)	279	989	1479	2484
12 (29 200)	8	55	110	349
20 (17 500)	(0.04)	1	3	20

[1] Number of groups (total population: 350 000 pregnant VDT-operators/year) in parentheses.

Annex 3 Table 2.   Calculated number of groups which will be expected to have a frequency of congenital defects higher than 35%, with variations due to different assumptions.

Assumed group sizes[1]	Rates of congenital defects in all VDT-exposed pregnancies		
	1.3 %	2.0 %	4.5 %
7 (50 000)	32	88	556
10 (35 000)	1	6	83
15 (23 300)	(0.01)	(0.01)	4

[1] Number of groups (total population: 350 000 pregnant VDT-operators/year) in parentheses.

W.H.O. Visual Display Terminals and Workers' Health